Pull the Plug?

By Patricia A. Smith

Cover design by Patricia A. Smith

This is the inspirational, true story of a mother who is devastated when her young, beautiful daughter suffers a massive stroke during a minor surgery to correct an irregular heartbeat. The surgery left her in a coma, quadriplegic, and in the Locked-In-Syndrome (LIS).

The doctors warned, "If she lives, she will never recover, never walk or talk again. What you see now is all you will ever see. It would be the kindest thing to just let her go rather than be selfish and possibly keep her alive like this for years."

With her daughter's life in the balance, she has to decide whether to listen to the doctors or go with what her own heart tells her to do. Would it be more merciful to "pull the plug" and let her daughter go, or let her faith guide her through the healing process in hopes of a miracle?

Pull the Plug?

No way!

Proceeds from the sale of this book will be placed into a fund for Maxine's college education; also benefitting will be the American Stroke Association and each of the ten churches that were so dedicated in prayer for Dorathy.

The opinions and thoughts expressed within are my own and are not meant to imply other's views. Doctors' names and their staff have been changed along with the names of some acquaintances.

Pull The Plug?

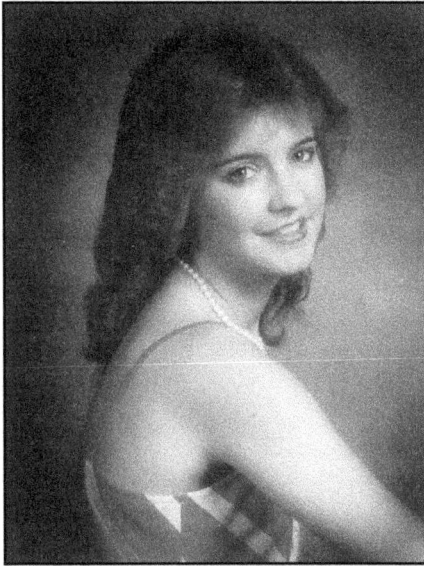

Dorathy

Courtesy of Lifetouch Studios, Inc.

I dedicate this book to my daughter, Dorathy. Her determination, courage, positive attitude, and internal fortitude for surviving such a real-life nightmare were astonishing.

Only God could love you more,

Mom/pas

Pull The Plug?

Seagull, Seagull

The watchful eye of the ever present gull constantly wondering what is in our skull. He is not a stranger; but a brother. We do as he does, analyzing each other. As to what he and we think. He has the control to come and go in a blink. The freedom of flight is in his soul, yet we are bound to the sand with no choice. I look and he looks, too. I turn for a second and the blink occurs. This travel he does is earth shattering, quick and in complete blurs. His thoughts transport him to another cloud. Things are thought not said alone. Seagull, Seagull with the power of flight we watch and wonder yet don't comprehend your plight. You're there yet out of sight, you do exist, yet not in the air; but you are the part of me that wishes for the freedom you have, ever cutting the winds of the world. I see you, I thank you. For you are me. Seagull of the wild, I wish I was just a feather on your wing. For I feel I am your child. I cannot fly with you in physical means, yet I am there by your side at every move. For you are me and I, you. When you bleed, I bleed. The pain you feel is in my heart. Seagull, Seagull you can never die for our minds are connected by the winds of time. For when you go into the end, I lose a most cherished friend. Seagull, Seagull please never part. For I am you and you --- me --- you exist as my light to see.

Patrik Hawk Stillwind, Author

Printed by permission

Pull The Plug?

If I Knew

If I knew it would be the last time
that I'd see you fall asleep,
I would tuck you in more tightly
And pray the Lord your soul to keep.

If I knew it would be the last time
I'd see you walk out the door,
I would give you a hug and kiss
and call you back for one more.

If I knew it would be the last time
I'd hear your voice lifted up in praise,
I would video tape each action and word,
so I could play them back day after day.

If I knew it would be the last time,
I could spare an extra minute or two,
to stop and say "I love you,"
instead of assuming you would KNOW I do.

If I knew it would be the last time,
I would be there to share your day,
well, I'm sure you'll have so many more,
So I can just let this one slip away.

For surely there's always tomorrow
To make up for an oversight,
And we always get a second chance
to make everything right.

There will always be another day
to say our "I love you's
and certainly there's another chance

to say our "Anything I can do's?"

But just in case I might be wrong,
and today is all I get,
I'd like to say how much I love you
and hope we never forget.

Tomorrow is not promised to anyone,
young or old alike,
and today may be the last chance
you get to hold your loved one tight...
so if you're waiting for tomorrow,
why not do it today?

For if tomorrow never comes,
You'll surely regret that day
That you didn't take that extra time
For a smile, a hug or a kiss
And you were too busy to grant someone, what
turned out to be their one last wish.

So hold your loved ones close today,
Whisper in their ear,
tell them how much
you love them and that you'll always
hold them dear.

Take the time to say "I'm sorry," "please forgive me,"
"thank you" or "it's okay."
and if tomorrow never comes, you'll
have no regrets about today.

Author Unknown

Acknowledgements

Thanks to Carol Williams for encouraging me to share my memoirs in hopes of helping others when told there's no hope for their loved one and they should just let them go.

Special thanks to Joyce Abbott, Ruth Bowen, Elizabeth Guilford, Leeoma Terry, and Joanne Urchisin, for all the hours (and days) they provided in making this book possible. Each thought and idea you contributed certainly added more interest to these writings. I appreciate all of your time and your enduring hard work. Thanks!

Most importantly, thanks to God our Father for listening to all those thousands of prayers for Dorathy and turning her around, allowing her to continue her life with her daughter, Maxine, her brothers, all her friends, her co-workers, and me.

Patricia A. Smith

Contents

*Trademark of Sheltering Arms
Physical Rehabilitation Center

Printed with permission

Pull The Plug?

Chapter 1

Code Neuro

"Code Neuro ... Code Neuro ... Code Neuro...," the intercom blared. Instantly, I knew that code meant there was trouble and with my daughter in the hospital surgical unit at that time, it scared me to death. With such severe code, it meant major problems. My daughter, who had been admitted to the hospital earlier in the day was having what we thought was minor surgery to correct an irregular heartbeat, due to Wolff-Parkinson-White Syndrome *(WPW).

I ran to the nurse's station and asked, "The coding is for my daughter, isn't it?"

Two of the nurses confirmed my worst fears. They came to me, consoling me in their arms, suggesting, "It would be best if you, your family, and your friends would move into a private waiting room down the hall."

As we were slowly walking to the new room, a set of double doors opened into the hallway directly in front of us. Nothing in the world could have prepared me to face what I saw next.

I looked at the patient on the gurney coming through the doorway, but not recognizing the patient I looked away.

Pull The Plug?

Suddenly I realized that the purple, swollen patient before my eyes was my very own daughter. She no longer looked like the beautiful forty-year old, petite brunette I had last seen going into surgery earlier that morning. *More detailed information about this condition is included at the conclusion of this book. "Oh, no. She has passed!" I exclaimed. I seemed to enter into a state of shock. I could not lose the daughter who had been so special to me from the time she took her first breath. Life without her would be unbearable. I didn't think I could continue to live if Dorathy passed.

Her friend Sandra enveloped me into her arms and held me. Sandra said, "She's okay. She hasn't passed. She's going to be okay." I knew Sandra was also extremely worried but felt she needed to console me. I was so distraught that I didn't believe her. I knew she was only trying to make me feel better.

Dorathy's cardiologist stepped forward and put his arms around me. He appeared to be very sad. He told me, "I finished Dorathy's surgery around 2:30 and everything seemed to be fine, I went on to my next patient. We are taking Dorathy for an MRI procedure now, and as soon as we know more, we will let you know."

"Go on and get the MRI started," I told him.

The time waiting for more information had a numbing effect on me. Could this really be happening, or was this just a nightmare? Time seemed to stand still. The next time I saw Dorathy, the MRI had been completed. She appeared more normal, as if she was just sleeping peacefully. She was receiving oxygen, and a ventilator helped her breathe. She no longer appeared purple or swollen.

After what seemed like hours, the neurologist finally returned and asked us to follow him to the Surgical Intensive Care Unit. Once inside, he pointed to the MRI on the computer screen and told us that Dorathy had a suffered a massive stroke. He said they didn't know for sure when it happened. It may have been during the surgery, or it may have been afterwards. A blood clot had gone to the worst possible place for it to strike: the brain stem.

"If Dorathy lives, she will never be anything more than a vegetable, will never utter another word, and will never take another step. She is a quadriplegic, paralyzed from head to toe, unable to speak or move. She will only be able possibly to blink her eyes. Dorathy is in the 'Locked-In Syndrome,' from which there is no recovery. She is in a coma and may never come out of it. The condition she is in now is as good as it will ever be." He continued, "We have only a small window of time to decide whether to let her go or not. I feel the kindest gesture we could make would be to just let her go."

"Please God, don't take my precious daughter," I prayed. I remember thinking the Bible says that God will not give you more than you can bear. Does He think I'm made of steel? How much more can I bear?

Pull The Plug? No way.

No one wants to hear those words, especially a mother who has cared for her daughter through childhood illnesses, through the loss of that child's father, through the birth of her child's daughter, and through the death of that child's father.

Dorathy had been okay at 1:30 p.m. and supposedly joked with the nurse. She also seemed to be fine at 2:30 p.m. when the doctor left her side. Then, at 4:00 p.m., she was in a coma and not expected to come out of it. Most neurologists say that if you can get a stroke victim to the hospital within three hours, the effects of the stroke can be totally reversed. She was already in the hospital.

"Why?" I asked. "Why didn't they try this procedure on my wonderful daughter?"

Pull The Plug?

Chapter 2

Day of Surgery

Prior to Dorathy's surgery, I had had a number of apprehensive feelings pertaining to the procedure and was not at all comfortable with the idea. I was afraid there would be complications. While knowing this was supposed to be a minor surgery, how could any surgery dealing with such a major organ be minor? Dorathy had not been feeling well for about two years. At times her heart would start racing, beating as if she had just ran in a marathon. This terrified Dorathy. She was afraid, that one day her heart would start racing and it would just explode. She knew she had to seek help; she had a daughter to care for.

Before she was hospitalized, I went to her house a number of times to help with the housework and to do the laundry.

One night as I was cleaning, Dorathy said, "Mom, do you want to hear some music?"

"Sure," I said. "That would be nice." Her selection of music had the tone of a funeral dirge; it was depressing; I could not control the tears as they flooded my face. Trying to keep my back turned to her, concealing the tears was almost impossible.

As I was leaving her house that night, we walked to the porch where we hugged and kissed goodnight. She said, "I love you, Mom."

I told her, "I love you, too, Dorth." (Dorth was a nickname I sometimes called her.)

It disheartened me to have to pull away and leave her. I noted as I drove down the street, that she stayed on the porch for as long as I could see her. I was extremely frightened that she might not make it through the surgical ordeal. My fear was of losing my favorite and only daughter. I had to pull off the road as the tears were impairing my vision and my driving might have endangered not only my life but the lives of many other people.

That night, I dreamed about my mother. She had died shortly after I had given birth to Dorathy. In my dream, my mother came back to life to be with me during Dorathy's surgery and to lead her home as she "crossed over." When I awoke, the dream had been so real I was extremely sad. Tears flooded my face. I was having such a hard time dealing with all this!

Dorathy called me two days before her surgery and asked, "Mom, would you like to meet me for lunch tomorrow at Joe's Inn?"

I told her, "I would love to, but I'm working." After hanging up the phone, I had second thoughts. I felt I had to spend as much time as I could with her, so I called back immediately and told her, "I changed my mind; I would love to join you for lunch."

During lunch, she shared with me that she wanted to make use of a Christmas gift card my friend Andy had recently given to her. The lunch was tasty, but I could not shake my sadness. When we finished, she returned to her work at United Parcel Service Freight (UPS Freight), where she had worked as a computer analyst for twenty-one years,

Day of Surgery

and I ran my weekly errands.

On the morning of February 28, Dorathy picked me up in order for us to ride together to the hospital. It was a cold, gray, wintry day. Who wants to have surgery on such a dull, depressing day? Her surgery was supposed to be a simple WPW procedure to repair a heart arrhythmia. During this procedure, the doctor would insert a catheter and destroy the extra conduction pathway of the ventricles to her heart. Her cardiologist had originally wanted to perform the surgery on February 21; however, as Dorathy's father had died a number of years prior on that date, she chose to have the surgery a week later. It was understood that she would spend one night in the hospital and go home the next day. I chose to stay the night with her at the hospital.

Driving into the hospital parking garage, I wanted to share with her my thoughts and fears pertaining to the surgery, but being afraid of scaring her, I said nothing. Later, I wondered if it would have made a difference.

Dorathy had preprogrammed her cell phone to text some twenty-plus friends, family, and coworkers telling them the surgery went well and that she would see them shortly. Little did she know that this message would never be sent.

As patients are usually advised to leave their valuables at home, I was surprised Dorathy was wearing her jewelry to the hospital. She wore a ring on each ring finger and one on her thumb that Patrik, her brother, had given her. Her diamond earrings were in her ears. When she went in for surgery, she gave me her purse for safe keeping. I placed the rings there, along with one her friend Larry had given her. The nurses taped her earrings to her forehead, which I thought was odd, but I suppose they thought they would be safe being with Dorathy. They were later given to me, and I placed them in her purse with her other jewelry.

When Dorathy and I walked into the hospital foyer,

my friend Andy was waiting for us. The three of us went upstairs to the Heart Catheter Department. As Dorathy was checking in with the admission person, she said, "I fear the outcome of the surgery because I'm a single parent of an eleven-year-old daughter, Maxine, and I don't like the possibility of leaving her without a parent."

When she had finished all her paperwork and we were sitting in the waiting room, Reverend Bill Martin, a minister from my church, West End Assembly of God, came to visit with us. We prayed together that God would guide the surgeon's hands and keep her safe. Dorathy thought I had gone overboard by asking the minister to come to the hospital for prayer prior to such a minor procedure.

Shortly after he departed, the nurse took Dorathy into the prep area. As soon as they had her prepared for surgery, the nurses told me, "You can see her before she's taken in for surgery."

I was frightened, but I tried to hide my feelings. She and I seemed to have the same awful thoughts. I believe we both had our doubts pertaining to the outcome of the surgery. Subsequent to our short visit, the nurses wheeled her away. Dorathy looked back at me with red, tear-filled eyes as if to say, "Mom, save me." Hating letting her go, I prayed, "God, please watch over my daughter."

While she was in surgery, her friend, Larry, waited with Andy and me. After work, her friends Sandra and Gina joined us. They never would have dreamed of what they were walking into.

Dorathy had been in surgery for quite some time when I became concerned. What was taking so long? We had not had an update at all. At 1:30 p.m. I went to the desk and asked to speak with someone. Finally, a nurse came out to give us an update.

She said, "Everything is fine. We went in on the right side of the heart, but the problem was on the left. The additional surgery will take a little longer. Dorathy is joking and carrying on. You may see her in a couple more hours."

Dorathy can recall that while she was still under sedation, Dr. Randolph asked the nurse "Is her mom still worried even after the update on her condition?"

I often wonder why the doctor didn't know where the problem was before he began the surgery. Having to go from the right side of the heart to the left not only took longer, but she had to have additional sedation for the longer period of time. The increased time and additional sedation increased the danger of the surgery.

Feeling somewhat comforted by the update, Andy and I told the nurse that we were going to eat and would return shortly. When we returned around 3:30 p.m., we waited for more news, but none came. I inquired again; again, nothing. A few minutes later, around 4:00 p.m., the news was blared out for all to hear. "Code Neuro ... Code Neuro ... Code Neuro."

Pull The Plug?

Signs of a Stroke

Call 911 immediately if someone is having these symptoms

Doctors say a bystander can recognize a stroke by asking three simple questions:

S*   Ask the individual to SMILE.

If the smile is lopsided, a stroke is likely to have occurred.

T*   Ask the person to TALK, to speak a simple sentence coherently (i.e., It is sunny out today.)

If the speech is slurred, a stroke is likely to have occurred.

R*   Ask him or her to RAISE BOTH ARMS.

If he or she cannot raise one arm, a stroke is likely to have occurred.

*NOTE: Another sign of a stroke Ask the person to stick out their tongue. If their tongue is crooked (if it goes to one side or the other), that is also an indication of a stroke

The American Heart Association

Printed by permission

Pull The Plug?

Chapter 3

Pull The Plug?

When Dr. Jackson gave us his prognosis of Dorathy's condition, I was devastated. This had to be a horrible nightmare. How could such a minor surgery go so wrong? I had lost my mom, dad, two brothers, four sisters, and two husbands, but I didn't believe I could live with the loss of my precious daughter.

It was hard to believe I was going to have to make phone calls to my sons, Jonathan and Patrik, informing them of such devastating news about their sister. When I called, and explained that the doctors were saying we should just let her go, they could not believe it either. They were both in a total state of shock and immediately left their home to be at Dorathy's side.

Patrik called Spencer, a dear family friend of many years, who lives in Charlottesville, Virginia and told him the awful news. He said to Spencer, "We need to get with Dorathy to pray for her."

When Patrik and Jenn, Patrik's fiancée, arrived in Richmond from Florida and Spencer arrived from Charlottesville, Virginia they immediately drove to the hospi-

31

tal where they prayed for Dorathy. Patrik said, "So many thousands of people were praying for Dorathy and that was a huge part of her healing. God was listening to all those prayers. That's the way miracles happen."

I thank God numerous times each day for giving her that ultimate gift of life once again.

Jonathan and Patrik came to be with me just at the time that I was faced with the decision of whether to "pull the plug" or not.

Dr. Jackson continued to say that we should let her go. He said, "It's the kindest thing you can do for her, or you can go the selfish route and keep her alive for you. She could possibly go on living 'as is'--in a coma for years."

While Dorathy was still in the Surgical ICU, another doctor made the same diagnosis as Dr. Jackson and repeated that the kindest thing I could do for Dorathy was to let her go. I still could not just give up on my daughter, a child who I carried in my womb for nine and a half months, who carried my blood in her veins and shared my DNA.

With Jonathan and Patrik only having one sister, they had always looked out for her, protected her, and they were extremely close. It was a great benefit to me to have them with me for support at such a horrific time in our lives. I prayed to God for guidance, asking that He not allow her to live in the same condition for years, but that He bring her back to us one hundred percent.

Patrik told me, "Mom, Jonathan and I are going to Dorathy's house to look for her Will, her Power of Attorney and her Medical Directive."

I told him that I would go with them to help find them since I thought I might have a better idea as where to look. We were so positive the legal papers were there somewhere, but we didn't find them. Being a military family, it had always been drilled into us the significance of having these documents. The importance of who would be appointed to carry out your wishes when you could no longer make the decision for yourself was also stressed. It must be someone who is fully trust-worthy and has that person's best interest at heart. I could not believe Dorathy would not have all her legal papers current and placed where they could be found. We had to find out if she had a safe deposit box where she may have placed them. Because I knew it would be noted on her tax records if indeed she had a safe deposit box, I contacted her CPA, who also did my taxes. He had worked for the same company as Dorathy for many years and knew her well.

When I talked with him, he said, "I just heard about Dorathy and I am so sorry. Come by and I'll check her return for any record of a safe deposit box."

When I arrived, he told me there wasn't any such record.

He had heard from UPS Freight employees that Dorathy wasn't expected to live and that eventually a copy of her last tax return would be a necessity in the handling of her finances. He tried desperately hard to be helpful, by making a copy of Dorathy's last tax return for me to give to her Power of Attorney, in case it was needed at a later date.

Dorathy's home computer was searched by an expert, and her supervisor at UPS Freight had her office computer searched in-depth for these documents, but still no luck. Nothing was found.

After all efforts were exhausted in the search for Dorathy's legal papers, we were introduced to a woman, who was a notary Jonathan, Patrik, and I signed the papers to appoint a Power of Attorney for Dorathy.

She told us, "The lawyer wouldn't make this a limited Power of Attorney, but I want nothing to do with any medical decisions. All medical decisions will be left to Dorathy's family."

I was grateful Maxine's Godmother agreed to take on the responsibility of Dorathy's finances in addition to seeing that someone was with Maxine before and after school and on weekends. I knew this situation was astounding to Maxine. As I was spending all my time at the hospital, friends and family were caring for Maxine. The judge agreed to give the Godmother temporary custody of Maxine. Our family had known since Maxine was born that if anything ever happened to Dorathy, Maxine's Godmother would be the one who would take care of her in order for her to have two parents.

While Dorathy was still in a coma, and the doctors were saying she would not recover, I certainly did not want to leave her. I wanted to devote all my time to Dorathy as long as I had that opportunity; I rarely left her side. The possibility that Dorathy might never wake up was terrifying. Comprehending losing my precious daughter was totally unthinkable. In prayer after prayer to God, I asked him to take me in her place. Being concerned about there being too many visitors, it was requested that only two people visit Dorathy at a time, only family and a couple of close friends. I called my place of work and told them about the terrible predicament Dorathy was in and that I wasn't sure when or if I could return. Of course, they certainly understood my need to be with my daughter.

Maxine needed her mom to take care of her. Maxine's father had passed away when Maxine was twenty-one months old; therefore Dorathy was her only parent--Maxine desperately needed her mother.

The second night after Dorathy's surgery, I was with her in the Surgical ICU and heard a female nurse call out to a male nurse who was assigned to care for Dorathy that night. She told him that there was an incoming call for him.

Pull The Plug?

When he answered the call, I heard him mention "Ms. Dorathy." I assumed it was one of the doctors calling to check on my daughter.

When he finished his conversation, I said to him, "I could not help hearing part of your conversation. It was concerning my daughter wasn't it?"

He said, "Yes, it was Visions of Life calling to check on the status of Ms. Dorathy because she is a donor." That call really troubled me. My thoughts were replaced with nightmares. I was frightened that during the night, some other patient's health might falter, and they would allow Dorathy to "fade away" in order to give her organs to someone else to save their life.

Later that night, the Visions of Life representative came to the hospital. He kept walking around in the Surgical ICU like a vulture circling its prey. This was an overwhelming experience for me. The following day, I spoke with the social worker for the hospital and shared my concern. She assured me, "We cannot and would not allow one person's life to "expire" in order to save another's life." She continued, "Visions of Life is not associated with our hospital; it is a separate entity."

I agreed to meet with the Visions of Life representative that day. He was very informative and explained in detail how the "Donor Program" works. He said, "One person's tissue and organs can save the lives of sixty-one other people." Having talked with him gave me a more comfortable feeling that they were not going to just let Dorathy "go" to benefit someone else.

It has been noted that:
One donor can save 7 lives through organ donation (heart, liver, pancreas, 2 kidneys,2 lungs) and enhance more than 50 lives through tissue donation..

An average of 17 people die each day from the lack

35

of available organs for transplant.

Make sure your family knows your wishes if you want to be an organ donor.

*More detailed information concerning this is included at the conclusion of this book.

Dorathy had always been thoughtful and caring of other people. For years, she had made a practice of donating blood as often as possible in order to help others. I knew that if she could save just one life, she would want to do so. To be able to save the lives of sixty-one other people would be pure heaven to her.

While Dorathy was in a coma, she never appeared to be in pain. I truly think that was God's way of protecting her. However, she constantly seemed to have some wild and strange dreams while in the comatose state. One of the night nurses in the Surgical ICU kept giving Dorathy morphine.

I asked her, "Does she really need such strong medication?" I knew that the longer she was on morphine, the longer she would lay there in a comatose state and that the pain medication could cause constipation, which would cause much discomfort.

Having worked as a private duty caregiver/companion, I knew the signs of a person in pain. She never had the furrow in her brow or frown on her face. She wasn't showing any signs of pain. As the nurse injected another dose of morphine, she said, "I just like to keep my patients comfortable."

Webster's dictionary defines morphine as, "The god of dreams." It is a drug derived from opium to relieve pain, and it has been proven to allow people to just give up and enjoy the dream world; it is also highly addictive.

Dorathy can remember, when she was still in a coma, she heard her doctor comment that he was afraid her brain might start swelling. "That scared me," she said. "I really started praying then." I wondered if that was why they gave her the morphine at first, to keep the brain from swelling.

I spoke with Dr. Randolph the following day during his rounds and asked him, "Does Dorathy really need such strong pain medicine? She doesn't appear to be showing any signs of pain."

He immediately nodded, saying "I don't believe she is in pain either. I will write up orders for the morphine to be discontinued." He did write up that order, and the morphine was stopped. I do not believe Dorathy would ever have come out of the coma if it had been continued. She would have stayed in the comatose state, still dreaming those wild and crazy dreams. I am so glad I made a point to ask about the medication.

One of the surgical nurses who assisted with Dorathy's operation came to visit her while she was still in a coma. She said to me, "All the nurses and doctors are concerned about Dorathy. We don't understand what went wrong. We wonder if a drop of blood formed a clot on a surgical instrument and it went into her blood stream." Dorathy says she remembers a couple of nurses discussing the amount of sedation they had given her.

After three days in the hospital and the morphine had been stopped, I thought that I had to get her limbs moving. I was determined my daughter was not going to end up as a vegetable; she would walk again! In order for her to walk, I knew she had to be exercised. I started thirty minute sessions, three times each day, working her arms and legs moving each joint up and down and side to side, to keep her from losing her mobility and flexibility.

We were told that music was helpful for people who had suffered a stroke; thus Maxine brought her CD player and some CDs to the hospital for her mom along with her iPod. The music was very soothing. We were careful to keep the volume low due to the fact she was still in the Surgical ICU.

In order to keep Maxine's life as normal as possible, Jonathan and his wife, Tracy, spent a week at Dorathy's home with Maxine making it possible for her to continue living in her home, sleeping in her bed, and going and coming as usual. Patrik spent the next week with her, and each week another person would stay with her. Angie, Maxine's Godmother, would usually take Maxine to her house on Friday and return her to school on Monday morning.

When our wonderful family friend, Tess, came to visit Dorathy in the hospital, she told us about a number of dreams her sister Karen kept having about Dorathy. At the time of the dreams, neither Tess nor her sister knew Dorathy was in the hospital, much less in a coma. Karen called Tess asking, "Is everything okay with Dorathy, Patrik's sister? I keep having dreams about her."

In Karen's first dream, Dorathy was in the hospital and told Karen, "Talk to me, so I can hear you. It will help me find my way back. I can follow your voice." In the second dream, Dorathy said, "Will you bring my girl to me?" After Maxine visited with her mom, Karen's dreams continued. In the third dream, Dorathy said to Karen, "Tell my girl to talk to me." Patrik suggested to Maxine that she should read to her mom. As a result, the next time Maxine came to the hospital, she climbed up into the bed with her mom and read to her; she also brought her iPod and played music for her mom. When the battery died, the iPod was taken home to charge it. In the next dream, the message was, "Where did the music go?"

In another dream, Dorathy said, "I'm tired of looking at those three spots on the ceiling." When this dream was revealed, we were all shocked as we looked up and saw the

Pull The Plug?

three spots on the ceiling of Dorathy's Surgical ICU space.

Tess suggested to Maxine that she make some drawings for her mother, she made so many the walls were covered in Dorathy's Surgical ICU section. Maxine and Dorathy would quite often lie in bed, side by side, enjoying the art display.

Wong-Baker FACES Pain Rating Scale©
Instructions for Usage

Explain to the person that each face is for a person who has no pain (hurt) or some, or a lot of pain.

Face 0 doesn't hurt at all. Face 2 hurts just a little bit. Face 4 hurts a little more. Face 6 hurts even more. Face 8 hurts a whole lot. Face 10 hurts as much as you can imagine, although you don't have to be crying to have this worst pain.

Ask the person to choose the face that best describes how much pain he has.

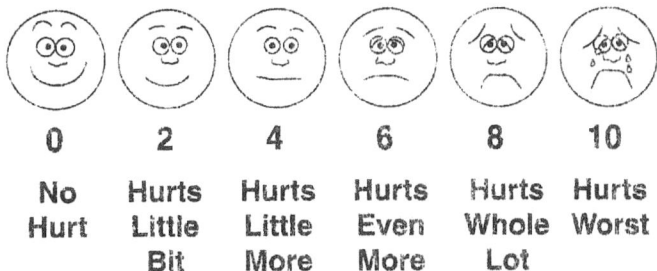

0	2	4	6	8	10
No Hurt	Hurts Little Bit	Hurts Little More	Hurts Even More	Hurts Whole Lot	Hurts Worst

Pull The Plug?

Chapter 4

Angels

My heart broke a little more as I stood at the foot of Dorathy's bed and observed the anguish on the faces of Jonathan and Patrik as they watched over their little sister. Here were two grown young men trying to hold back their ever-flowing stream of tears. This time when Dorathy needed help, they felt powerless. There wasn't anything they could do for her now. It was heart wrenching.

Early one morning, I was sitting in the Surgical ICU waiting room, while the nurses did their 7-8:30 a.m. duties, and a lady asked me, "Are you with the young lady who had the massive stroke?"

"Yes, she is my daughter," I replied. "We've been told the kindest thing we could do for her would be to just let her go."

"Don't be too quick to make a decision. There's no hurry." She told me about someone she knew who had gone through the same type of stroke as Dorathy a year prior. That person had returned to work and was now walking, talking, and has very few problems.

Her doctors had told her family the same as Dorathy's doctors were telling us, "Just let her go."

Again she said, "Take your time; there's no rush; give her time to heal." Was this an angel sent to me by God? I had never seen her before, nor have I seen her since.

As Andy and I entered the elevator a few hours later, a doctor, who I had never seen before, joined us. "How's your daughter?" he asked.

I replied, "She's not doing well. Her doctors are telling us to let her go, that it would be the kindest thing we could do for her."

He made the same recommendation as the lady in the waiting room; "Take your time; let her heal, and then decide what to do. There's no rush." It was as if God was sending these people to guide me, to help me make the right decision.

I have never seen either of these concerned and sincere people again. I do believe they were placed in my path to lead me, to help me with the toughest decision in all my life. I often think of these two wonderful people and would love to thank them in person for their helpful advice. They emphasized that there was no rush to decide, when many of the doctors were in a hurry for a decision to be made.

On the third day after Dorathy's surgery, the hospital chaplain took Maxine, Angie, and I into a private conference room to explain to Maxine what was going on with her mom. She asked her if she was aware of what was happening to her mom.

"I know my mom is very sick."

The chaplain then told her, "Maxine, your mom is extremely ill. There is a real possibility your mother won't get any better and you may lose her."

Maxine didn't say anything, but it was obvious that she was very sad and hurting inside. It was impossible to hide the facts from her. She and her mom had always been inseparable.

Angels

Dorathy's doctors, the chaplain and I thought we should let Maxine know what could be a real possibility, in case her mom didn't survive.

Maxine just sat there, as if she was thinking very deeply, curled up in a protective ball in her chair. Angie and I each had an arm around her. My heart was breaking for my only grandchild.

Maxine later cried and said, "First I lost my dad, and now I'm losing my mom." Although it appeared that Maxine just wanted to be alone, her friend, Carson stayed by her side to console and comfort her.

It was an ironic state of affairs; Dorathy and Maxine each losing their father at a very early age. Dorathy's father had passed away while on active military duty a few months prior to her eleventh birthday. Maxine lost her father a few months before she turned two. Now, nine years later, she simply could not lose her mother.

When Maxine was younger, she would see her schoolmates from day care being picked up by their fathers and would cry saying, "I want a daddy." At other times, she would pretend to call her dad on the phone and once she even said, "Well! He hung up on me." I didn't want to have her feel that parental absence all over again.

Three days after the surgery, Dorathy was no longer on morphine, and we began to see before our eyes a miracle in progress. Her eyelids began to flutter, much like the wings of a beautiful butterfly, but the eyes stayed closed. After thirty or forty-five minutes of fluttering, the left eye opened a fourth of the way. As time passed, the eye would open to approximately half way, then three-fourths, and finally opened all the way and stayed open. A short time later, the right eye started opening in the same way, a little at a time with the same fluttering action. When the right eye had completely opened, it looked faded, as if she was blind. It was sad to think she might be blind in that eye, but we were excited to see her beautiful eyes once, again open. We thanked God that at least she was still alive.

Her left eye seemed to focus on an object or a person; however, the right eye appeared to look off to the side, blurred and unfocused. This was the first physical evidence to back up our feelings that the doctors could be wrong in their diagnosis. To us, this was real progress, but the news didn't excite the hospital staff. They said, "Families just see what they want to see, but what you see is all you will get." Our family; however, was just in awe of her newly found abilities.

Dr. Randolph said, "The muscle in the right eye is weak due to the stroke, but it will be okay." We were delighted when, later in the day, it did catch up with the movement of the left eye. Although Dorathy's eyes were now open, she was still a quadriplegic and in the "Locked-In Syndrome." Dorathy was now able to communicate by blinking her eyes to "yes" and "no" questions. Jonathan initiated this procedure with her, and we were all excited about our new way of communicating with her. Jonathan told Dr. Randolph about Dorathy's latest development. Dr. Randolph said that it was just a reflex making her blink. Jonathan then told Dorathy to open her eyes for "yes" and to close them for "no." As the doctor looked on, Jonathan and Dorathy proved their point that Dorathy knew what she was doing when she would blink or close and open her eyes for "yes" and "no" questions. Dorathy was mentally alert and remembered everything as soon as she came out of the coma.

But her doctors were still skeptical, saying, "She'll never be better than what you see now. What you see is all you'll get." These were disappointing words, and I kept hearing them over and over again. This was my cherished daughter whom I loved so deeply and felt so close to. She just had to get well! They were still telling me I needed to let her go. This was not what I needed or wanted to hear. I was devastated! Hurt! Sad! Angry! But it made me even more determined not to give up!

The physical therapist, occupational therapist, and speech therapist would come by to see Dorathy and would just walk away without attempting to help her in any way. They had, evidently, seen her chart with the written report that Dorathy was beyond help.

After her physical therapist, Jim, saw how hard I was working on exercising Dorathy's limbs and how determined I was, he brought me some drawings of exercises for her. It was obvious however; that he didn't think it could possibly help. I continued working with Dorathy morning, noon, and night. Her limbs were already becoming stiff. I repeatedly worked her finger joints, wrists, arms, elbows, toes, ankles, feet, knees, legs and head ... morning, noon and night, every day. At first it felt that if I moved them too much, they would break. They were heavy, much like dead weight. It was all I could do to lift them. I knew her doctors thought I was wasting my time exercising her, but I knew I wasn't! I knew my daughter could pull out of what she was going through with God's help. She was like her mother. She was strong, and she was determined. We were not about to give up.

The doctors, nurses, and therapists would come by as I worked with Dorathy on her exercises. Some of them would just shake their heads and walk away. They couldn't believe I thought I could possibly help her. Other people would comment to her, "You are certainly lucky to have such a dedicated mother who is so much help to you." This comment usually brought the responses of a twinkle to her eyes or a "rolling of the eyes." She still could not speak, so all of her expressions had to come from the movement of her eyes. It always made us laugh when she would respond in that way. A few weeks later she was able to shrug her shoulders as another way of communicating. Then she could almost carry on a conversation by the rolling of the eyes and the shrugging of her shoulders. To me this was another sign that the doctors were mistaken in their prognosis. More precious signs of life!

As with most mothers, my love for Dorathy made me want to do all within my power to help her in all possible ways, almost as if I was on auto pilot. My reward would be to see my daughter move her arms, legs, hands, feet and head on her own. I would be fulfilled when she could turn her head, talk, walk, eat, drink, and laugh again. We often take these actions for granted, not thinking about how a tiny blood clot going into the brainstem can incapacitate some-one for life or snuff that life right out of them.

Dorathy later told me that Dr. Randolph would sometimes come into her space in Surgical ICU while she was in a coma, assuming that she didn't know he was there. He would just stand near her bed and sob. She said, "He would never say anything but quite often would stay as long as what seemed to be fifteen minutes crying." Dr. Randolph was very compassionate, and I know he felt sorrow for the situation. It was such a sad predicament.

————————

The doctors suggested that Dorathy should have a tracheotomy (trach) to replace the ventilator. They said that, if need be, they could always reinsert the ventilator. The doctors explained, "When Dorathy is taken off the ventilator, she can continue to breathe for ten to fifteen minutes. She might even survive for two or three days." The nurses had cut back on Dorathy's dependence on the ventilator, and she was breathing almost completely on her own.

It was also suggested that Dorathy should have a peg tube (feeding tube) as she was unable to swallow, so all her nutrition and hydration would enter her stomach directly. The Peg tube is inserted through a small incision in the stomach. The idea of a feeding tube was extremely scary for me. I had known numerous other people who had used them, and every one of those patients had died. So, to me, this new surgery was a sign that she might not live. This was becoming scarier as the days passed.

During this time, her brothers and I decided that we could not make these major decision for her, since Dorathy knew everything that was going on and could answer "yes" and "no" questions, we decided that we should ask her what she wanted to do. We agreed that Jonathan should be the one to ask her.

As we circled around her, Jonathan asked, "Dorathy, would you want to continue to live if you have to live as you are now?"

With the closing of her eyes, she told us "No." Then, to make absolutely sure she understood us completely and we understood her blink, Patrik asked Dorathy the same question again; again, her answer was "No." Her brothers and I decided to give her doctors the go ahead to do the trach and the feeding tube.

I prayed to God, saying, "If you are going to take her 'home,' please take her prior to her having to endure the pain of the two surgeries."

I asked Dorathy if she had asked God to forgive her for any sins in her life. She answered with her eyes, "Yes." I also asked her if she was ready when God was ready to take her home. Again, her eyes told me "Yes."

I thought the two surgeries would be more complicated than they proved to be. While they performed the surgical procedure in her area of the SICU, the doctors allowed me to stay in the room with her. It only took fifteen to twenty minutes for both procedures.

Now with the feeding tube in place, Dorathy was able to receive her nutrition. (Ill people need more food than a healthy person in order to recover). I had thought she was receiving her essential nutrition and hydration through the intravenous fluids, but while the fluids were supplying her with her required hydration, she was not getting her needed daily amount of fat, iron, vitamins, and protein. She had not had anything to eat since February 27, and this was March 10. That was a total of eleven days.

Dorathy and I prayed together. I suggested, "I know you can't speak, but we can still pray. I will say the words, and you can pray silently, or you can pray using different words." And so, we prayed.

Doctor Jackson was still saying, "She'll never speak another word." It was so difficult talking to her and thinking she may never again be able to speak. It broke my heart.

Dorathy cried a lot, and we didn't know why. She didn't appear to be in any type of pain. We felt helpless, not knowing how we could comfort her. Maybe she was missing her daughter. Maxine came to the hospital often and would, at times, quietly climb up onto the bed and lie with her mom, sharing some artwork or homework. It always delighted Dorathy to have Maxine by her side.

When Dorathy began responding to her exercises, her physical therapist, Jim, and his co-worker started to show more interest in her. They ordered braces for her hands and arms as well as for her feet and legs to help adjust them back into a normal position rather than in the "Locked-In" position that had caused them to turn inward. They also started exercising her and allowed her to sit on the side of the bed.

The doctors and nurses were also beginning to spend more time trying to help. They would often walk up to the foot of her bed and touch her foot saying, "Can you feel that?"

She would blink "Yes." They were checking to see if she had any feelings in her right side, because the stroke had affected her right side much more than the left.

They would then walk up a step closer to touch her

leg and again ask, "Can you feel that?"

Again, she would blink "Yes."

As they continued their exploratory research, moving up the right side of her body, they would touch her arm and again the question I know Dorathy had heard at least hundreds of times, "Can you feel that?"

Again, she would blink "Yes." At a later date, she would just roll her eyes. After a while, when the nurses and doctors would come into her room, she seemed to know what their little "game" was going to be. She would look at me with an expression in her eyes as if to say, "Well, here they go again with their little games; time for more blinking."

An acquaintance of Dorathy's said that I treated Dorathy like she was a four- year old. Of course I was protective. At this point, she couldn't do anything a four-year old could do. I tried to assist her in every way possible, by spending every single day in the hospital with her, for the three months she was hospitalized.

Pull The Plug?

Chapter 5

UPS Freight Delivers

Dorathy's employer, the UPS Freight Company, formerly known as Overnite Transportation, was absolutely wonderful and very supportive throughout this tormenting experience. The employees came to the hospital while Dorathy was still in surgery and were with our family during the crucial meeting in the hallway. They stayed with us during Dorathy's initial MRI procedure and when Dr. Jackson gave us his bewildering diagnosis.

When the UPS Freight "Family" heard the news of Dorathy's plight, it seemed every employee who had ever met her wanted to be at her side. They converged on the hospital. Some of the nurses designated the SICU waiting room as "Dorathy's UPS Waiting Room." Families of other patients made their way to a waiting room down the hallway in order to allow Dorathy's family and friends to be together near her.

While Dorathy was still in a coma and the doctors were saying she would not recover, we had been told that patients with brain injuries should not be over stimulated by having too much company, I was afraid she was getting exhausted from so many people being there, even though she was comatose. It was suggested that visitors be limited to family and a few friends. I was trying only to do what was best for my daughter's health. I wasn't willing to leave her side.

Nance, a supervisor at UPS Freight, designated a room at the UPS office building as "Dorathy's Room." This was a room for people who were having a difficult time dealing with Dorathy's condition to grieve and to pray for her. There were lots of flowers and Bibles in the room, and counselors were made available for anyone who needed them. The love and care of Dorathy by her co-workers and friends was very evident. Everyone was exceptionally thoughtful and interested in her well-being. They were such a comfort to our family, even in our state of grief and confusion. With so many of Dorathy's friends at our side, we knew she was loved by them. Numerous co-workers told me (between sobs) how much Dorathy meant to them saying, "If it hadn't been for Dorathy training and helping me, I wouldn't have a job with UPS Freight today."

Schedules were made up immediately at UPS for those who would prepare food for our family each night. The food was delicious and so beautifully prepared, as if it had been designed by professional chefs. We went to my house to rest and have dinner between 7:00 and 8:30 p.m., during the time the SICU was closed to all visitors in order for the nurses to prepare the patients for the night. At that time Eve and the UPS employees would deliver our wonderful hot meals. We ate and returned to the hospital. It was truly a blessing to have such nutritional hot meals prepared when we arrived home. We didn't have to shop for food or prepare it. They brought so much food every night that I finally had to ask them to cut back. The next day, I opened my front door and what did I see? A UPS delivery truck! My first thought was, "Oh, my! Was this more food?" However,

UPS Freight Delivers

it was just UPS making their regular deliveries.

Dorathy's friends were very thoughtful. I thank them, and I thank God for each of them. True to their profession, they really did deliver in our time of need! May God richly bless each of them.

Pull The Plug?

Chapter 6

Therapists

Approximately three weeks had passed since Dora-thy had been admitted to the hospital, and the doctors were still not giving us any hope. I was not giving up on my amazing daughter. I continued to exercise her each morning, noon, and night. Up to this point, she had not helped me at all; however, one day, it finally became evident that she was putting forth effort to help me move her left leg. Patrik said that he, too, had felt her trying to help him with the exercises. Now, each time the leg was bent or moved, she was helping with that movement. I was elated and shared the marvelous news with Dr. Randolph.

Still, he said, "It's just a reflex. It is normal for the family to 'think' they feel or see something as a sign their family member is improving. Naturally, they want to believe the patient is recovering."

I didn't say any more about it, but I knew that move-ment was there, and I knew it meant she could do much more. I wasn't about to give up on her.

We had repeatedly been told by numerous doctors "To let her go"; "What you see is all you will ever get"; "It's the kindest thing you can do for her"; "She'll never be any better than what you see now"; "If she lives, she'll never be more than a vegetable"; "She'll never utter another word, and she will never take another step." I heard those statements so often that I would even hear them in my sleep. It affected me and made me feel as if I was already in mourning. I hated seeing my beautiful daughter in such a helpless state.

A few days later, Dr. Randolph came in to make his rounds. While he was standing beside Dorathy's bed, she raised her knee up from the bed and into the air. She then let it lay back down on the bed. Her doctor was astounded. He asked me, "Did you see that?" His eyes were about to pop out of his head. He was so excited. As soon as the left leg was on the bed, she would raise it again and again. Dr. Randolph was in shock. He just couldn't believe it.

I told him, "I've been telling you for days that she has been helping me with her exercises." Everyone was excited. They all found it hard to believe that a person who was not expected to live or to ever move her limbs again was now helping to exercise those limbs. No one now thought this was a reflex. God, we thank you!

Angie thought I was staying at the hospital too much. She stated, "I feel we've had too much mother-daughter togetherness."

She had never had children and didn't know how it felt for a mother to be so close to losing her only daughter. Dorothy still was unable to help herself in any way. An infant can cry when hungry or when it's too hot or cold and can kick the covers off when needed. Dorothy couldn't do any of those minor tasks; someone had to help her, and that someone was me. The nurses were certainly helpful, too. They did everything they could to help, but they were overworked and understaffed as all hospitals seemed to be.

Therapists

After the doctor saw the movement in Dorathy's leg, he brought in a physical therapist, Jim, and his assistant. They started really working with her stiff joints and muscles. An occupational therapist was even helping, teaching her how to use different aids to help in everyday situations. Dr. Randolph called Dr. Khokhar from another hospital to ask him if he would come in and interview Dorathy concerning her going into the rehabilitation program at the Johnston Willis Rehabilitation facility. After Dr. Khokhar came in to evaluate her, he stated, "She is not capable of doing six hours of rehabilitation each day, and that's what we require. The stroke made her very weak. She first needs to work on building up her strength and her muscles. I think she would benefit from going into therapy at Retreat Hospital Rehabilitation now. After a month there, she should be strong enough for our rehabilitation program at Johnston Willis Rehabilitation Hospital."

Dr. Khokhar contacted a registered nurse named Sandy, who was Assistant Director for complex care at Retreat Hospital. He asked her to come in and evaluate Dorathy, and she did so. Sandy was a wonderful, kind, considerate, and professional person. She talked with Dorathy and had her do a number of different exercises. She wanted to find out exactly what Dorathy was capable of doing and what her needs were. A patient had to have difficulty in five different areas to be considered for the Retreat Rehabilitation Program. Dorathy certainly fit into that category.

When she finished her evaluation, I wanted Sandy to know how important it was for Dorathy to get into a good rehabilitation program. I had taken my latest framed, five-by-seven school picture of Maxine to the hospital in order for Dorathy to always have Maxine nearby. I picked up the picture, handed it to Sandy and told her, "This is Maxine, Dorathy's 11-year-old daughter. Maxine needs her mother at home, and I need my daughter. We need your help in order to get her into a good rehabilitation program." The tears started flowing, not only from my eyes but Sandy's too. Although we still had to have approval from the insurance company, she immediately approved the move into Retreat Hospital Rehabilitation.

Dorathy's therapist brought her an alphabet communication card. She still could not speak, but she could blink her eyes. When she wanted to tell us something, we would point at the different letters on the card until she would blink. Frequently, by the time a sentence was spelled out, we would forget what the first letters were. This was confusing for her, so we decided to write out the words as she chose the letters. That helped. Her spelling ability was not hindered by the stroke. She also knew how to use sign language, but none of our family knew how to converse using sign. It was wonderful experiencing such a remarkable development; things were slowly but surely improving.

She decided she wanted a bedside commode. She still couldn't get out of bed, but she wanted it and she got it. She never used it, but again … she got it. At that point, I think if she wanted the moon, all she would have had to say is "I want the moon," and the staffs' quick reply would have been, "When?" They were certainly doing everything in their power to accommodate her.

Around the time of Dorathy's early rehabilitation efforts, Andy found a brochure in the hospital on "The Power to Overcome" and gave it to me. It was from Sheltering Arms Physical Rehabilitation Center. They had a seminar scheduled for May 15 pertaining to inpatient rehabilitation. I made it a point to attend.

In the hospital, I met a young man named Ed who told me about Sheltering Arm's Physical Rehabilitation Center. His mother had a massive stroke much like Dorathy's and had benefited greatly from all the therapy at Sheltering Arms Rehabilitation Center. She was now walking a mile a day and was almost completely healed.

Ed took me to Sheltering Arms to meet Dr. Silver and some of his staff. Dr. Silver explained to me the Bioness Technology treatment for the legs, arms, and throat. He gave me a folder of information about Sheltering Arms Physical Rehabilitation Center, a folder about Bioness, and a DVD for me to give Dorathy. He wanted her to actually see how the Bioness system worked. The Bioness treatment can reduce complications such as atrophy and muscle spasms, while increasing the range of motion and blood circulation.

Ed offered to go with me to the hospital to see Dorathy. He thought it might help her to understand everything better if it came from a source like his mother. He explained the Sheltering Arms Physical Rehabilitation program and the Bioness treatment to her and told her how much it had helped his mother to recuperate.

I had seen "The Power to Overcome" billboards and had watched the ads on TV about the Sheltering Arms Physical Rehabilitation Center. Andy had given me the brochure, and now I had met a man who was telling me all about what a Godsend Sheltering Arms had been to his wonderful mother. It was as if God was saying, "Open your eyes; I've sent you numerous people to help. Use what I've sent you!" I was so in hopes Dorathy would be receptive to this latest idea of treatment.

Hanna, one of Dorathy's many nurses, anointed Dorathy with oil to help her and bless her in her recovery. Patty, another nurse, was such a gem and did everything within her power to assist Dorathy, often doing things for her beyond the call of duty. She and some of the other nurses knew it had been cleared by Dorathy's insurance company for her to go into a nursing home, and they were not at all pleased with that decision.

Pull The Plug?

When I was informed that the insurance company wanted Dorathy discharged from the hospital and sent to a nursing home, I was appalled. I had no idea she would be discharged in the condition she was in. She still could not do anything for herself; she couldn't go to the bathroom, couldn't shower, couldn't walk, talk, eat, or drink. They wanted to send her away from the hospital in that condition?

The hospital's social worker gave me the names of a few nursing homes which were on the list Dorathy's insurance company would approve. Maxine, Angie, Andy, and I looked at a few of the homes. Some of the homes would not even consider taking Dorathy due to the fact that she was on a ventilator and had a peg tube.

"What do you think of that one?" I asked Angie, after looking at the first one.

She said, "I think it is okay; what do you think?"

I replied, "I think it's a dump! My daughter would not put me in a place like that, and I'm not about to place her there either. I will take her home and take care of her." And I did just that.

Dorathy's physical therapist and her nurses were all upset to think she might be going into a nursing home. They knew she wouldn't get the rehabilitation there that she so desperately needed. Each of them was doing all within his or her power to persuade the doctors to tell the insurance company that Dorathy had to go into rehabilitation in order to fully recover. One kind person even made a note of an increase in Dorathy's temperature in order to keep her in the hospital one more day to give us more time to work on a rehabilitation program.

When I called the insurance company telling them I was Dorathy's mother and I needed their approval to get Dorathy into rehabilitation, they told me, "I can't discuss this with you. We have already approved a nursing home for her."

Therapists

I told them, "Then I would like to speak with your supervisor." The supervisor took my call. I told her "My daughter is young and intelligent. She has worked for UPS Freight twenty-plus years. She has an eleven year-old daughter and is a single parent. She needs your help to get some badly needed rehabilitation. She needs more than what a nursing home would provide for her. If she goes into a nursing home, she will receive very little rehabilitation. The rehabilitation program may cost your insurance company more at first, but it will be for a shorter period of time due to the fact she would be in a nursing home forever." A lot of people I had worked with on my job as a private duty caregiver/companion quite often had to go to a nursing home after a long stay in the hospital. These were older people in their eighties and nineties. They were not planning on being rehabilitated to return to work, and they received just enough help to be able to walk in their homes. Dorathy's goal was to return to work.

The supervisor said, "I will check on this and get back with you." I wasn't going to give up at this point; my daughter's livelihood was at stake.

I talked with Dr. Randolph about the quandary. He contacted Dr. Khokhar, and Dr. Khokhar spoke with the insurance company. Dr. Jackson, the neurologist, also got in touch with the insurance company on Dorathy's behalf. The CEO of the hospital was contacted by one of my former clients asking for assistance in getting approval by the insurance company for Dorathy to go to Retreat Rehabilitation Hospital.

John Sebastian, Dorathy's supervisor at UPS, had told me, "If there is ever any way I can be of help, please do not hesitate to call me." I called him! We needed all the help we could get. I was determined not to take a chance on her being placed in a home other than her own. I told him about the insurance company wanting to dismiss Dorathy from the hospital and send her to a nursing home and also told him about the run around I was getting concerning the approval from the insurance company for a rehabilitation program.

He said, "Let me make a few phone calls to check on this." He seemed to have gotten the insurance company on the ball because the next day Dr. Randolph called telling me that the insurance company had approved of Dorathy going into Retreat Rehabilitation Hospital. I thanked God again and again! I was so relieved.

Dr. Randolph said, "I don't know who you called or how you did it, but whoever it was, it worked. Even the CEO of the hospital was in on this move."

I told him, "If it had taken another twenty-four hours to get what Dorathy needed, I would have had the Governor in on this move."

Dr. Randolph said, "I believe that!"

Everyone continued their efforts in helping Dorathy do anything and everything she wanted. They could not seem to help her as much as they would have liked. The nurses, doctors, and therapists were practically running over each other to do for her. It was as if a new "Star" was born. (Dorathy's middle name is "Star.")

Andy noticed that all of the patients names were listed on a bulletin board at the nurses' station and told me, "They've put a red heart beside Dorathy's name." None of the other names were accompanied by a red heart. We thought it was so sweet that they would do that. They always did treat Dorathy special (probably because she was in such poor health). We later learned the red heart meant Dorathy was their only donor in that section of the ICU--the "one" who still wanted to help other people.

Chapter 7

Memories/Times of Concern

I remember when Dorathy was just three months old, her father, Max, a career military man, was transferred from Fort Carson, Colorado to Hanau, Germany. On this tour, the military would not allow us to take Dorathy out of the United States until she was six months of age. As a result, Dorathy, her brother Patrik, and I stayed in Arkansas with my parents until we could join Max in Europe. My father tried to talk me out of making that long trip across the "Pond." I was, after all his "baby." (Dad and I had always been extremely close) I know it bothered him to see me go so far from home. None of his other children had ever been out of the United States.

When Dad would ask me, "Are you sure you really want to go so far away from home...and with those babies?" Mom would not even give me a chance to answer his question; she would interject and come to Max's defense by saying, "Now, don't try to talk her out of going. Her place is with her husband."

A few days after the military sent our airline tickets for us to join Max, Mom asked Dad to take her shopping for Dorathy. Mom had never driven and had no desire to do so. She bought the most beautiful little black patent leather, hard-soled shoes with an ankle strap closure and small pink flowers centered with a pearl on the toe. I told mom, "Dorathy can't even walk; she doesn't need shoes." I thought little bootie-type socks would be more comfortable for her and easier for me to keep up with on such a long trip. After all, I was embarking on a three thousand mile trip with two children under the age of three.

Mom insisted, "Our baby cannot leave our homeland and go into a 'strange' country without shoes on her feet."

I gave in. Dorathy wore her new shoes to that "strange" country. She always loved those shoes and kept them for years after she outgrew them. I was thankful I gave into mom's request concerning the shoes. Tragically, my mother suffered a heart attack and passed away six weeks after our departure from Arkansas.

There had been a few times in Dorathy's life when I had been extremely worried about her. I recall that, even at the age of two, Dorathy was so petite and precious. We lived in Europe at the time, and my sister Helen arrived to spend six weeks with us. We wanted to make sure she had an enjoyable visit, so my husband, Max mapped out a vacation for us. We were first to go to Dachau, Germany, a former concentration camp, then into Austria, Liechtenstein, Switzerland, France, Andorra, Belgium, and Holland before returning to our home in Hanau, Germany. It was a wonderful trip. We had a great time and Helen was delighted to be with us. Our children adored her, as did she them.

However, upon our return home, Dorathy became ill with flu-like symptoms and was running a high fever of 102 degrees. The military doctor prescribed an antibiotic for her. After only one dose of the medication, she became completely engulfed in a red rash that covered every inch of her flesh. I immediately called her doctor, and he said, "Throw that medicine away and bring her to me now!" He later told us, "One additional dose could have been fatal." She was allergic to the antibiotic. She was so ill that we were afraid for weeks we were going to lose her. We made a bed for her on the couch, and Helen and I would take turns sitting beside her, bathing her with a cool wash cloth to keep her fever down. After she finally began to recover, she was again up and about, feisty as ever. She was still the apple of Max's eye.

Another time that I was so frightened was when Dorathy gave birth to her daughter, Maxine Nicole. I've always believed that what goes around comes around; therefore, I should not have been hurt when Dorathy didn't want me with her when she delivered her baby. My mom had been with me when my son Patrik was born. He was a breach birth, and I had to have early induced labor. It was a rough and dangerous delivery (back in the old days). When I survived it, along with a healthy, eight-pound boy, everyone was shocked, including the doctor. He said, "I don't know where in the world that baby came from." I had only a slight weight gain and I was very petite.

When it came time for Dorathy to come into the world, my mom was afraid I might have another rough delivery. She wanted to be with me. Mom had never flown in her life, but I was her baby, the youngest of her twelve children. She had purchased some new clothes and accessories and was packed to travel from her home in Arkansas to our home in Colorado Springs, Colorado. Breaking the news to her that Max wanted it to be just him and me at the hospital for the delivery was hard for me to do. Knowing how much it hurt her bothers me to this day. It makes me sad and brings tears to my eyes to think about it.

I sat in the waiting room as Dorathy gave birth, occasionally making my way back within sight of Dorathy's suite. I knew she was having a rough time by all the activity. The nurses were rushing in and out of her delivery suite to acquire additional equipment such as forceps and bringing in another doctor. I prayed over and over, again. Finally, it was all over. Mom was fine, but Maxine, my grandbaby, had a broken collar bone from the forceps being used to assist in the delivery. Mom and Dad were certainly elated and very proud of their little bundle of joy. She was a cutie! I waited at the nursery window for my first view of my grandbaby. The nurse brought in an adorable baby wrapped in a pink blanket. The baby had an abundance of black hair just like her daddy. There was enough hair on her head for three or four babies. I just knew that had to be our Maxine Nicole. I was wrong. It wasn't her.

Soon after that, another nurse brought in a baby. She, too, was wrapped in a pink blanket (because she was a girl). She also had dark hair and eyes of brown. The look on her face seemed to say, "Hey, Gran. It's me!" And, it was indeed our Maxine Nicole.

On the day of their dismissal from the hospital, a nurse took mother and baby to the car in a wheelchair while Bob retrieved the car. As we waited for the nurse to check the infant seat and to make sure "Mom" was buckled in, I looked up toward the sky to thank God again for being there for us, for protecting our family through rough times. At that moment, I saw the most beautiful double rainbow. To me, I felt that was God's way of telling me everything was going to be okay. I thanked Him.

Patrik and Dorathy were always close as children, and anyone could easily see when one hurt, the other hurt. One day, after their father had passed away, I came home from work. They were fighting and fussing like brothers and sisters do. I said, "Patrik and Dorathy--stop it! I just came home from work, and I do not want to listen to that."

Memories/Times of Concern

Dorathy started crying and said, "But mom, I love him." It was so precious.

————————

When Dorathy was young, we had a small white poodle. We affectionately called him Snowball. One day, we took Snowball to have him groomed. Upon our return to pick him up, he was asleep and could not be awakened. He had been sedated to keep him calm during the grooming, and we had to leave him there overnight. When he awoke the following day, we took him home, but it did take a few days for him to recover. Dorathy's saga brought back the memories of Snowball's dilemma, a very sad time.

Pull The Plug?

Photos

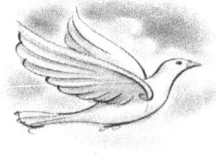

All photos copyrighted by Patty's photography,
unless otherwise noted.

Pull The Plug?

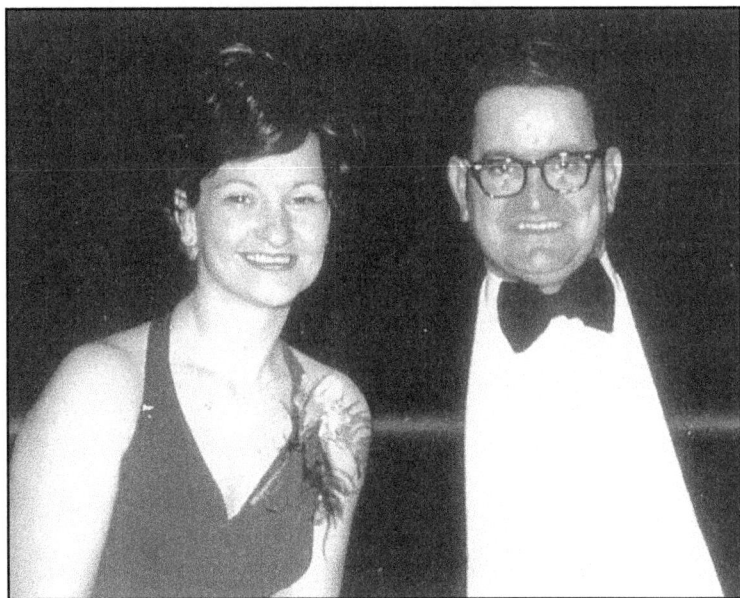

Patricia & Max – Dorathy's Parents

Pull The Plug?

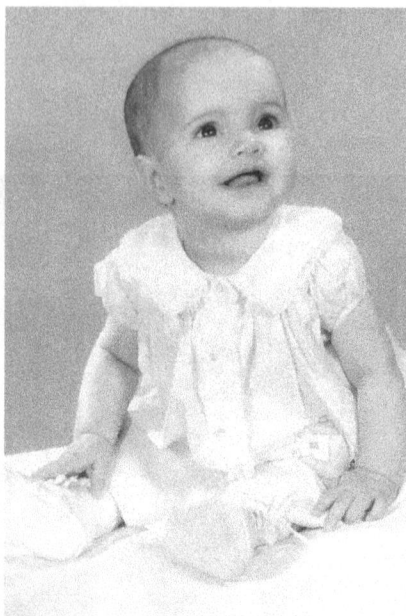

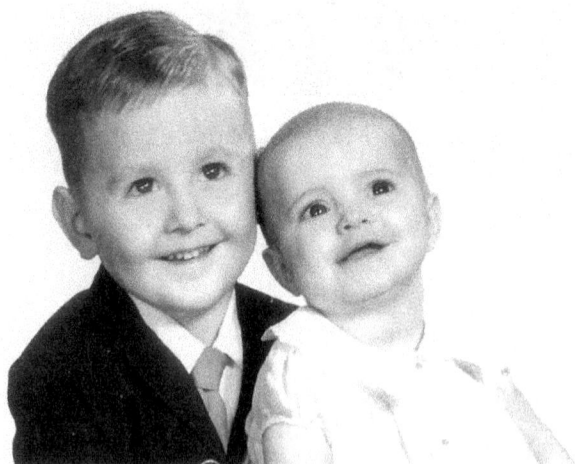

Patrik & Dorathy
Photo Courtesy of Gardner's Studio

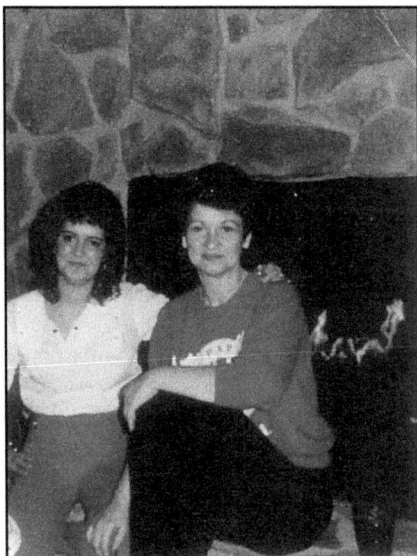

Dorathy & Me

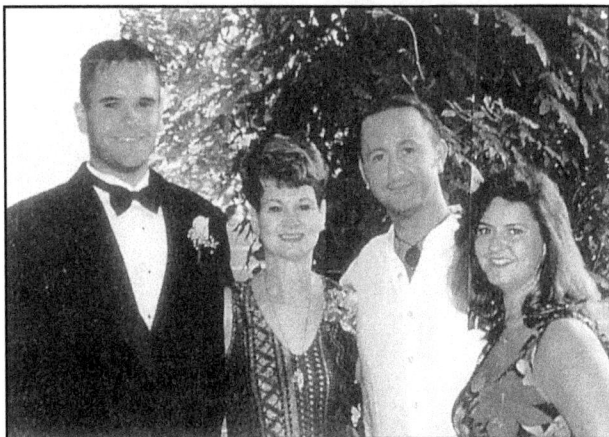

Jonathan, Me, Patrik & Dorathy

Pull The Plug?

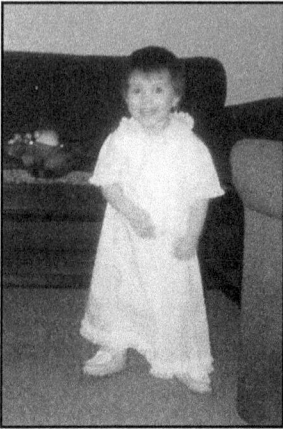

Dorathy – In Europe

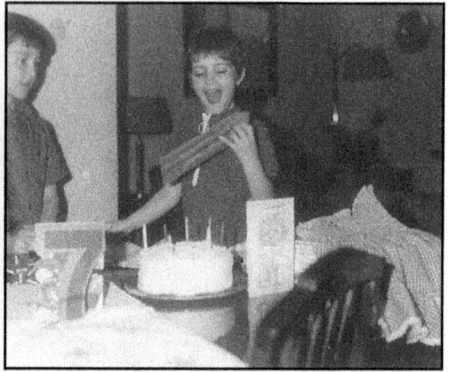

Patrik & Dorathy
Her 7th Birthday

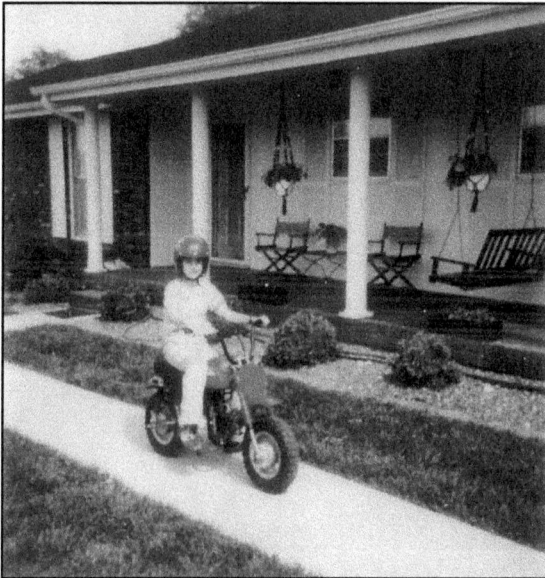

Dorathy – Her 12th Birthday

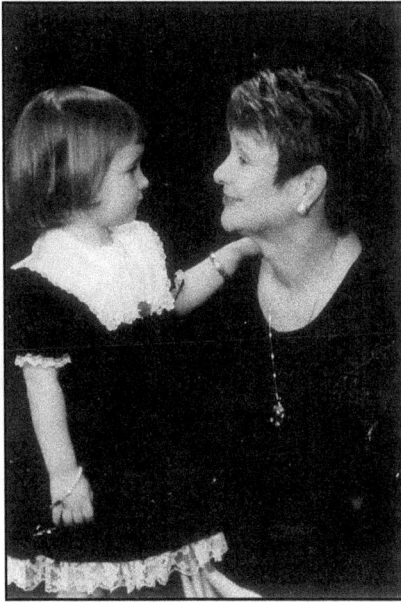

Maxine & Me
Courtesy of SEARS Studio

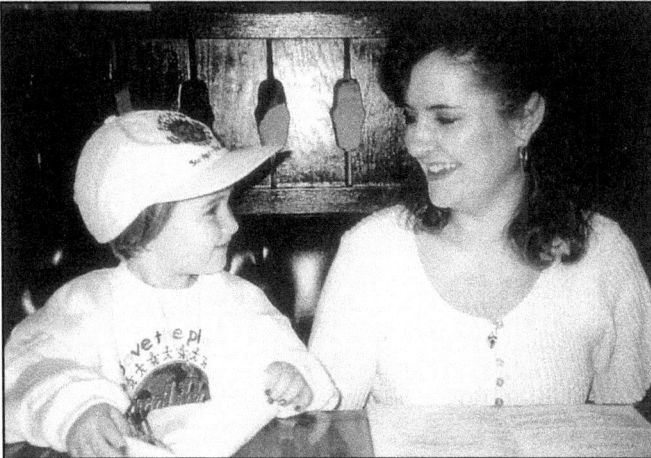

Maxine & Dorathy

Pull The Plug?

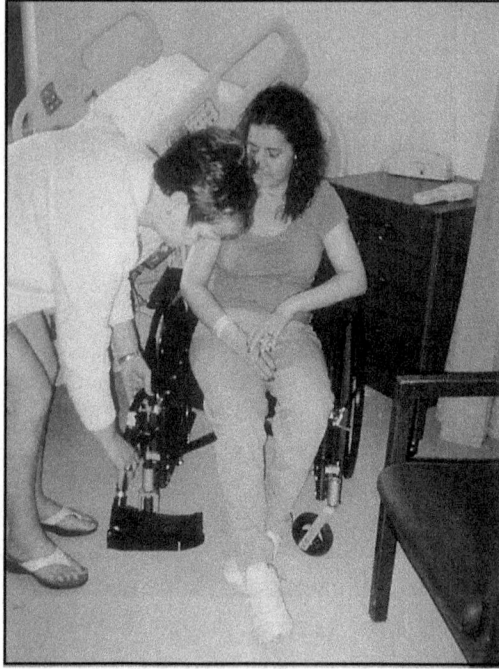

Leaving the hospital, Dorathy & I

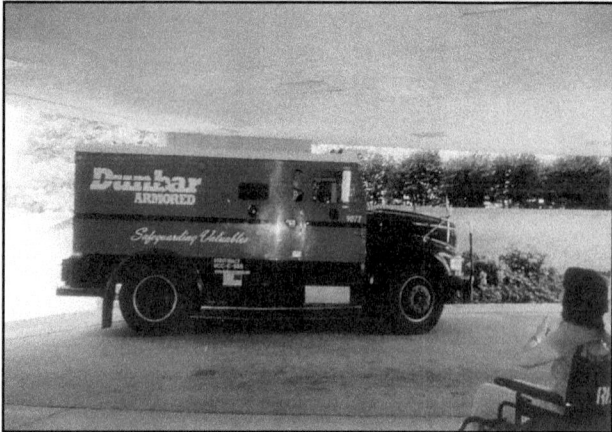

Dorathy pretending to thumb a ride from the
Dunbar Armored truck as she leaves the hospital.

My sisters – my rock
during Dorathy's long three month hospital stay
Loretta, Wanda, Retha & Me

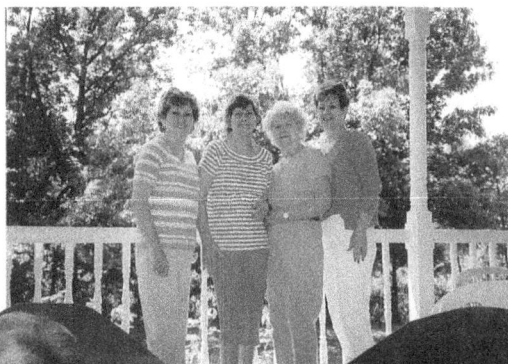

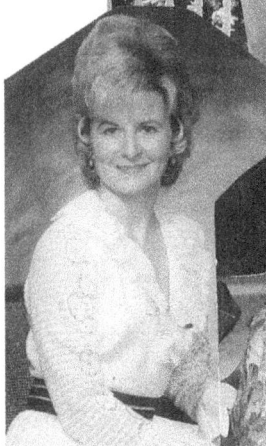
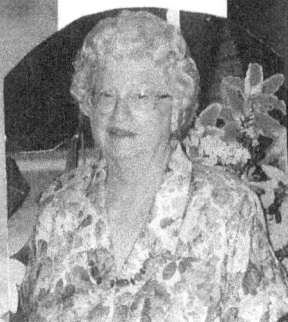
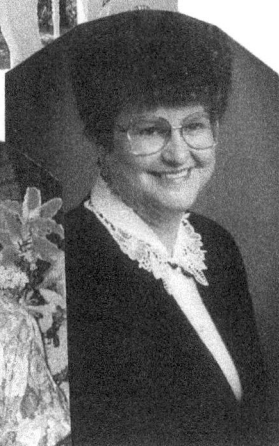

Helen   Vernice   Linda

Photo courtesy of   Photo courtesy of
Turi Photography   Gardner's Studio

Pull The Plug?

Chapter 8

Retreat Rehabilitation Hospital

I was delighted that Dorathy had been approved to go to Retreat Rehabilitation Hospital. We were feeling extremely optimistic and expecting the most out of their facility. Meeting Sandy, the RN from Retreat Hospital, had enhanced our optimism, and we felt that this was surely a major step in the right direction. Everyone there was wonderful.

Dorathy was very pleased when she heard she was being transferred to the Retreat Rehabilitation Hospital, but she was concerned as to how she would be transported to the new facility. The hospital's social director told her, "Leave that to us. We will take care of moving you." Dorathy was still unable to use a wheelchair. She was taken by ambulance to Retreat Rehabilitation Hospital on March 28, one month after her admission into her first hospital.

Dorathy was placed in the last room at the end of the hall, the furthest distance possible from the nurses' station. I feared her ability to communicate with the nurses. Happily, the nurses rigged the call button with a special device to make it work for Dorathy. If anyone was in her room visiting, she would form her mouth into a pucker to tell the visitors to be quiet. Then she would manage to push the newly rigged call button. The nurse would respond over the intercom to her call and ask Dorathy what was needed. When there was no response she would come in to check on Dorathy. She thought this was such a funny way to get the nurses in her room. Some of the time it seemed like a game with her. She couldn't control much, but she was the master of that little call button. She seemed to relish that idea.

The room seemed to be very bare of furniture. It must have been a double room at one time but was now a private one. The lack of furniture was probably to make room for all the different equipment the patients with special needs would require.

When the air conditioner in Dorathy's room malfunctioned, they moved her into another room which was much closer to the nurses' station. This was much more comforting to both of us. I felt she was safer.

And again ... I said, "Thank you, God!

When Dorathy complained, it wasn't that the personnel did anything wrong. She only wanted to double the amount of therapy she was getting. Using her alphabet card she spelled out, "I'm bored. I want therapy twice a day. I want to get better." Of course, she was granted her wish. I'm sure the hospital had to check with her insurance company to find out if they would cover both a.m. and p.m. therapy sessions, but they did so without complaint. The extra exercises certainly helped make her stronger and better fast. Plus, it was something to do rather than just lay around in the hospital room. The double therapy sessions exhausted her; however, she continued to push herself hard. She was so determined to get better more quickly.

Teasingly, I had told her that as hard as I had worked

with her, the first word out of her mouth must be "Mom." Sure enough, one day as I was straightening her room and putting away her fresh laundry, I thought she was asleep, my back was to her. All of a sudden she said, "Mom." I turned around to make sure of what I had heard. We were still being told she'd never speak. As I turned around, she said again, "Mom, please." What more beautiful words could a mother hear? I was overly thrilled, tears filled my eyes. I couldn't have been happier or more relieved. Of course, at that time it wouldn't have mattered what word she spoke. The fact that she could now speak was wonderful. It seemed as if God was right there in the room with us. It was another magnificent gift from God.

"Mom" had not been her first word as a child; "Dada" had been her word of choice then. I was so overwhelmed, so happy to hear my daughter speak. With this, it was more proof that the doctor's prognosis was wrong. It was beginning to prove that they could be wrong about so many other things. Could she possibly get the use of her voice back completely? Could she get the use of her arms and legs back? Could she walk again? Could she work again? Could her life return to one-hundred percent? Well …I only knew that God had His hand on Dorathy. She would make it!

At the end of March, Dorathy's doctor ordered an EEG and another MRI to be performed on her. The EEG was completed with no problem. Yet when it was time for the MRI, she started crying uncontrollably. She cried hard and for so long that it was impossible to complete the screening. I had asked about going with her for the MRI, and the nurses had said, "There is no need for you to go. It won't take long and we will return her to her room." After Dorathy started crying, a nurse came to me and told me what was transpiring.

She said, "She's crying so hard that we had to cancel

the MRI."

"Will you take me to her?" I asked. After all she had endured, I was terribly concerned about my daughter.

She said, "Come with me."

I did as she said. We went downstairs in one elevator, and Dorathy was brought up in another at the same time. When we arrived in the area of the MRI procedure, Dorathy was gone! We couldn't find her anywhere, and it frightened me. Finally, we went back to her room, and she was there. The nurse had given her a shot to calm her down and she was fine.

Her nurse asked me, "If we reschedule the MRI for another day, would you go with her and hold her hand, just to let her know you are with her?"

I told her, "Of course, I will."

On April 1, Dorathy was given a shot to keep her calm during the MRI procedure and, with me by her side, was taken into the procedure room for another attempt with the MRI. They placed a chair for me close enough to the machine that I could lay my hand on Dorathy's leg and she would know I was there. She was too far into the machine for me to hold her hand. The fact that I was with her and the shot she received earlier seemed to have a calming effect on her.

The noise from the MRI machine was unbelievable. It was clinging and clanging so loudly every minute she was in it. How she tolerated it I don't know. I was praying all of the time she was encapsulated that she wouldn't start crying again and that she would keep her eyes closed as they had told her to do. Everything went fine, and the MRI was completed. It would have been interesting to see how the new results compared with the one on the day of the stroke, but I didn't get to do so.

The hospital beds at Retreat Rehabilitation were special beds which were built for special-needs patients. The beds could be maneuvered into numerous positions. The nurse put Dorathy's bed into the position of a recliner; this position helped her to be able to sit up and to build up her strength and to re-learn to control her head. After she was able to sit up, she became stable and could control her movements much better.

She was then measured and evaluated to determine her needs for a power chair. When the long-awaited time came for the power chair to arrive, she was elated. It was a real "Mercedes." It had all the bells and whistles you could imagine. The chair was a bright burgundy red and was custom built especially for her.

The controls were built onto the left, which was her stronger side and worked with just a slight touch. At this time, she did not have good use of her left hand and virtually no use in her right hand. The power chair had a support to rest her head in order to keep her head from falling to one side or the other, and a tray with an indention for a cup was detachable. The chair would recline and also raise or lower with just a touch of a button.

Using a "hoyer" lift, a body harness was placed on Dorathy, it was attached to a lift that would extend over the bed and hook onto the body harness, she could then be lifted out of the bed by the nurses and placed into a wheelchair or another chair. This was a Godsend. To know that with help she could now get out of bed and move from place to place in her wheelchair by herself was such a relief to her. She was so happy.

At first, she wasn't the greatest driver. She kept running into walls, furniture, and doorways, but after a few days, she got the hang of it and would speed down the hallways, bounce in and out of the elevators, and outside she would go. Nance, one of Dorathy's supervisors at work, thought the power chair was so sporty looking that she brought some racing strips to place on the chair. That was just too cool.

Pull The Plug?

One day, the Retreat nurses could not find Dorathy. They searched the entire hospital for her. Finally, they found her outside in the flower garden where she was just sitting, enjoying the sights, the fresh air, and the freedom of being able to go to places by herself without any help or an escort.

"It's okay to go outside as long as you stay on this block where the hospital is. You can't go any farther." The nurse told her, "Once a man was so excited when he got his power chair, he went up the street to Carytown and got stuck in the doorway of a store. The business called the hospital; we had to go there to rescue him."

Dorathy answered, "I'm not going to take my power chair to Carytown. When I go to Carytown, I will be walking." She still could not speak clearly but most everyone could understand her. Maxine was almost as excited about the new power chair as her mom was. She loved to ride in it around the room. She also enjoyed escorting her mom in the chair around the hospital.

———————

When Dorathy was first admitted to SICU, the nurses had taped Dorathy's respirator tubing and mouthpiece to her face in order to keep it in place. When it was removed, the glue residue from the tape stuck in Dorathy's hair. It made it almost impossible to comb or brush. For weeks, I just worked around it when I would do her hair. I tried to remove the residue using ice, but that didn't work. I decided to cut it out, but I couldn't do that without cutting her hair. She couldn't talk, but she knew what I was doing. She would dart her eyes around and frown, watching as closely as she could as I cut the glue from her hair. I still was unable to remove all the glue. A few days later, her friend Larry tried the same procedure thinking she would never know. She did! She had a note placed on her bulletin board: "Do not cut Dorathy's hair."

———————

Retreat Rehabilitation Hospital

Dorathy's doctor ordered a Barium swallow test for her. This test can be used to check the upper digestive track and to observe the soft palate for difficulties in swallowing. She did not pass the test. The muscles which control the soft palate were still not working efficiently. She would have to keep the feeding tube in place until those muscles were working properly; otherwise, food or drink could go down the wrong tube and cause her to develop pneumonia. Her doctor said, "If Dorathy contacts pneumonia, she could die easily since her system is not strong enough to sustain her now. It could be a year or longer before her system is strong again." She seemed disappointed since she had been looking forward to once again having some real food and drink. It was sad for me to see her hopes dimmed another time. I was so in hopes everything would go smoothly; she had been very patient, but there wasn't anything anyone could do to speed up the process.

Maxine had an early birthday party and wanted to have a sleep-over. Quite a few of her friends were invited to her house for the party which had an Asian theme. The decorations were beautiful. Oriental lanterns were hanging from the chandler over the dining room table and of course the plates, glasses, chopsticks, and napkins all matched. There were small gifts for each child. The food was also oriental and was hungrily eaten by all.

What a scene they made with the cake. They fed each other and had a lot of fun, but what a mess they made! Tracy, Teresa, Jacqie, Angie, (all friends of Dorathy's), and I stayed there for supervision and help. Dorathy had always been there for Maxine, so it was obvious that Maxine missed her mother not being at the party; they were so close.

Maxine received a trampoline, and the children loved it. Dorathy had sent orders home from the hospital, "Only one child at a time can be on the trampoline." They all tried their best to get past that rule, but too bad. No luck. The sleep-over was a huge success.

April 14 was Maxine's actual date of birth. Maxine bought a small cake and took it to the hospital; she and her mom could then celebrate her birthday together. Dorathy stuck her finger in the icing and tasted it. This made them both happy.

From his home in West Palm Beach, Patrik came to Richmond to visit with Dorathy on April 15. He called when he arrived at the hospital, and I handed Dorathy the phone. He told her he was in the parking garage. Dorathy was sitting in her power chair when she took his call. When she hung up the phone, she said in her best speech, "Come, Mom, and follow me." I followed her to the elevator, through the long hallway, and when we were approaching the sharp turn into another long hallway, I glanced at the round ceiling mirrors which were placed there to see if someone was coming in the opposite direction. I saw Patrik and Spencer coming down the hall about to turn the corner. I stayed back and let Dorathy continue by herself, allowing the petite little female roadster in her racy power chair to get to her destination. Spencer and Patrik both moved to the side of the hallway as she approached them; they did not realize the little roadster was Dorathy. When she was even with them, she stopped. They were shocked that this could be Dorathy. They were laughing and overjoyed to see such an improvement and her running around by herself. We all had a big laugh. Neither of them had seen her with the power chair before. They were expecting her to be much like they had last seen her in bed, although they knew she had the power chair.

UPS Freight employees often came to visit Dorathy. In a mid-April visit, three or four of the employees came in not just to visit, but to bring Dorathy a laptop computer.

Retreat Rehabilitation Hospital

She was so excited, like a child in a candy store. Her hand extensions (her computer) were back in place. She was extremely happy. When I walked into her room, she and her co-workers had formed a circle of chairs; there were two men and a couple of women spending their lunch hour all busily working to get Dorathy on line. What did she ever do without a computer at the tips of her fingers? Her hands were still not working properly; however, the left hand was making some progress. She didn't use the laptop a lot at first, but she slowly eased into it. I believe the computer being there encouraged her to work her hands more than if she hadn't had access to it.

At that time, the right side of her body just didn't want to cooperate, it was much slower than the left. The right hand had a long way to go before it would be ready for computer work.

The nurses said Dorathy was the best patient in the hospital. She never asked for anything unless she really needed it, and she never forgot to say "Thank you." Even when she couldn't speak, she would manage a hand signal or something to relay a message of thanks. Dorathy never seemed to get upset about having to stay in the hospital for months with no anticipation of how long the stay might be. She never had pity parties like some patients. Nor did she ask, "Why me?" God was never questioned.

One day at Retreat Hospital, Dorathy awoke from her nap. I was straightening her room and putting away the fresh laundry with my back to her. She said, "What in the world happened to me?"

I told her, "They said you had a stroke. I doubt if we'll ever know what really happened."

I mentioned to Dorathy that my friend Leeoma had also had a stroke. I told her how she had fully recovered. She rarely has any effect from it. Dorathy asked me to talk with Leeoma and ask if she would come to the hospital and talk with her concerning her recovery. Leeoma was happy to share her success with Dorathy, and listening to Leeoma seemed to encourage her. I believe it gave her more hope for the future.

While Dorathy was in rehabilitation, she needed a manicure and a pedicure. I only had pink nail polish with me so I used that. It really was a beautiful hot pink color. Every time someone would come in, they would notice how nice her nails looked. Because Dorathy was still in the "Locked In" situation, she could not move her hands into her sight to view her nails. They would exclaim, "Oh, what beautiful pink nails!" Dorathy would have a bewildered look on her face. She knew she never wore pink polish. She always wore fire-engine red. After a few days of so many "well intended" compliments on the pink polish and all the bewildering looks from Dorathy, I decided the pink polish had to go. Maxine brought her mom some brownish-red polish, and I re-did the manicure and pedicure. Still, it didn't look like Dorathy's nails--although it was better than the pink. Later we were able to find the fire-engine red nail polish. We re-did her nails; this time it looked like Dorathy's nails again. It was beautiful. After that manicure, Gina, Dorathy's co-worker and friend, brought her a manicure/pedicure gift set and she took over the job of giving Dorathy her manicure and pedicure. She enjoyed Gina's pampering. It was amazing to see how much this simple deed lifted her spirits.

As I watched the Retreat team of physical and occupational therapists work with Dorathy, each re-learned achievement was such a big deal, both to Dorathy and me. When an infant starts to feed itself or it takes the first steps, it is wonderful, but when you've been told your grown child will never be more than a vegetable, will never take another step, will never utter another word--- seeing the doctors proven wrong certainly convinces you that God still has some major miracles in his bag. Thank you God! As she accomplished those goals, it brought tears of happiness and much gratitude to me.

We had no idea as to what extent Dorathy would recover; I thought I would be taking care of her for the rest of our lives. I started shopping for a house for all of us. Maxine and I looked at a large, beautiful townhouse. The unit was a good size for the three of us, and I thought the large master suite with a large bath and whirlpool on the first level would be great for Dorathy. She would have access to the entire first level in her wheelchair. Maxine and I would each have our bedrooms upstairs, and there was a loft area, perfect for another sitting area for Maxine and me, giving Dorathy more privacy downstairs.

After checking out the townhouse, we went to the hospital to see her mom. Maxine said, "Gran, show mom the picture of the house we looked at, the one you may buy for us."

Angie was in the hospital room and said, "I don't think that's something we need; Mom, Grandma, and granddaughter all living in the same house."

While Dorathy was in Retreat Hospital, her therapist suggested that it would help Dorathy to have some high-topped tennis shoes to support her ankle better. She was still wearing a leg brace on the right foot, since the Locked-In-Syndrome had left her leg turning inward. After some searching I found some high-topped navy blue tennis shoes and purchased them for her. They were ugly, and Dorathy was forever making fun of them. She did; however, wear them. She would do anything if she thought it would help her recover faster.

Pull The Plug?

When Dorathy completed her rehabilitation at Retreat Hospital, she was happy to be transferred to Johnston Willis Rehabilitation. I think she realized it was another step forward to a full recovery. The staff had been wonderful and had worked extremely hard to help her in every way they possibly could. She hated leaving her power chair behind, it was like leaving a good friend, but she was not allowed to take it with her. She said her good-bys and thanked the staff for their exceptional help. They had been outstanding to her.

When we were given Dorathy's prognosis, at her first hospital, I requested a floating air mattress be placed on her bed. I knew this was going to be a very long hospital stay. The air mattress would prevent her skin tissue from breaking down and causing bed sores. Dr. Randolph wrote up the order for the mattress to be placed on her bed. With each move Dorathy made from SICU, Vascular ICU, Retreat Rehabilitation Hospital, and to Johnston Willis Rehabilitation, she always had orders for the air mattress. Never once did she have a bed sore while spending three months in the hospital.

Chapter 9

Johnston Willis Rehabilitation Hospital

Dorathy was transferred to Johnston Willis Rehabilitation on April 23. She had been in the hospital about two months. Dr. Khokhar was the first doctor to be called in to evaluate her for rehabilitation. Dr. Khokhar had told me, "I will hold a bed for Dorathy. When she finishes her rehabilitation at Retreat and is strong enough for more extensive treatment at Johnston Willis Rehabilitation, she will have a place to come to." Dr. Khokhar was one of the doctors who had also helped Dorathy get her insurance company to approve rehabilitation.

When Dorathy arrived at Johnston Willis Rehabilitation, she was greeted with a manual wheelchair. She was extremely disappointed after having had such a deluxe model power chair, one that was exceedingly easy to use. Her arms and hands were not strong enough to move the manual chair. She was unable to maneuver the chair and had to be pushed everywhere. She hated it. It made her too dependent upon other people. Maybe they thought it would make her stronger if she had to work the chair manually, but she simply could not do it. She was not capable of getting from one point to another and had to have assistance to move across a room.

Her therapy was started immediately, and that delighted her. The staffs of therapists were very professional, and we could tell that they were interested in their patients and in their work.

A few days after Dorathy's arrival at her third hospital, she was quite surprised to have two of her doctors from her first hospital to come for a visit with her. Dorathy thought it took a lot of nerve on their part to come by after recommending pulling the plug, saying that she would never be more than a vegetable and that she would never take another step or speak another word.

I could never thank God enough for the wonderful miracles He has performed. I give Him all the praise for bringing Dorathy through such a terrifying time. I have never prayed so hard for so long in my entire life. God was listening to all our prayers. He was working with us. Knowing our God could bring Dorathy back one-hundred percent was reassuring.

All of Dorathy's senses were intensified. Her sight, smell, and hearing were better than they had ever been. She was still using the feeding tube; therefore, it couldn't be determined if her taste had been affected. Her doctor said that in time her accelerated senses would return to normal. We were thankful there seemed to be no memory loss. As soon as she started talking, she could be asked for the phone numbers of her co-workers, friends, or family and could recite those numbers automatically without hesitation.

Andy was so very patient. He stayed beside me every minute I was at the hospital. When I was not at Dorathy's side, I was constantly thinking and worrying about her. He wanted to make sure he was nearby in case Dorathy's health deteriorated. I knew he believed, as did the doctors, that there was no chance she could improve, but he stayed to support me and to be there for Dorathy. I do not know how I would have made it through all those days without him.

I called my place of work and told them about the terrible predicament Dorathy was in and that I was unsure if or when I'd be able to return. I had to be with my daughter. After Dorathy had been in the hospital a couple of months, I told Andy, "I think you should make a life for yourself without me. I know Dorathy is going to need me for a long time."

During physical therapy on April 25, Dorathy walked across the room twelve feet with the assistance of a board laid across the top of her walker, much like a shelf. She was so proud of herself. A few days later, her hand was swollen, but no one seemed to know why. No one thought it was anything to worry about. They said maybe she slept on it wrong and maybe the circulation had been cut off. Dorathy seemed depressed and she wasn't feeling well. She was, however handling the situation better than I could have. It had to be devastating to be a young forty year old women with a daughter of eleven and all of a sudden to be stricken with a stroke. Not knowing what her future would be, how Maxine would get along, and how she would be left financially, and if she would be able to return to work, were all questions that must have loomed in her mind. Maybe that was the reason she sometimes cried.

The next day, the hand was better; the swelling was gone; she was feeling great, and she was in great spirits. She walked thirty feet with the board. The following day she really went to town. She walked 150 feet--and her strength was improving each day. Her physical therapist was overjoyed with her. Each time Dorathy made a major accomplishment, she was overjoyed and so was I.

_____

Pull The Plug?

The first of May, Dorathy's brother Jonathan and his wife, Tracy, came to visit her. They were amazed at the improvements she had made since they last saw her shortly after her operation in March to apply the tracheotomy and feeding tube. It was such a dramatic improvement-- almost like seeing someone else. Everyone was elated to see each other.

Also on the first of May, Dorathy made her first phone call. A nurse was walking in the hallway and Dorathy managed to get her attention. She asked her to dial my number, and the nurse was happy to assist her. When I answered the call, she said, "Just called to say that I will talk to you later."

I said, "Okay, I love you. Bye." It was a heart lifting, precious message. Again, it made me feel great. This was another first.

Later that week, Dorathy was in the bathroom when I arrived at the hospital. When she came into her room and saw me, she exclaimed, after clearing her throat, "Hey Mom!" She put a lot of energy into those two words, but they were spoken so clearly, more so than any words she had spoken up to that point. With most of her speech, a person had to really listen closely to understand each word, possibly asking her to repeat the words again; but at least--she was talking. Her doctors had said she'd never utter another word. She was doing more than uttering.

Dorathy discovered on May 10 that the insurance company wanted to send her home. She had made a lot of improvements, but she still had a tremendously long way to go. They said, "At this time, in-home therapy is the best treatment for Dorathy." Her therapists doubled their sessions with her to make sure she was as fully rehabilitated and her muscle strength was as strong as possible before she left the hospital. They really pushed her and also themselves.

Notes from Dr. Victoria Tate's Stroke Seminar at Sheltering Arms Physical Rehabilitation Center

* Music without words is great for relaxing.

* Don't be embarrassed by your actions, such as laughing, crying, or saying silly things at odd times.

* If you want to walk - walk!

* If you want to use your hands - use your hands!

* Personality changes- -especially toward the person closest to the patient. The patient may hurt them; they may take out their frustration on the person closest to them.

* Patients want to control everything and everybody. They not only want things done for them, but they want it done, NOW!!

* Six months--the patient will make the most improvements during this time.

* Rehabilitation - only half-way there. Like a half-baked cake.

* Move !!! Do not sit around

Pull The Plug?

I attended the Sheltering Arms Stroke Seminar which was very informative for patients who had had a stroke and for their family members. The seminar helped me tremendously. Had I not had the information Dr. Tate supplied, I would have been lost as to what to expect next. I might have thought I was the only person who had ever experienced these changes. Some of the information seemed far reaching at the moment but later they were right in line, as to my daughter's actions. When these changes started, it hit me like a bolt of lightning. I couldn't believe my daughter, who I had always cherished, would turn against me.

Dorathy's therapist told me that Dr. Khokhar mentioned giving her Botox to relax the muscles in her ankle and foot. Botox is a muscle relaxant. Some doctors use it to treat facial muscle spasms. After having recently read in a medical journal that Botox can go into the brain stem and cause symptoms like a stroke, I was concerned about the procedure, especially after what Dorathy had been through in the last three months. I asked Angie her opinion concerning the use of the Botox treatment.

She said, "Oh, I think it's great. I think she should have it." When, I voiced my concern to the doctor; he said he wasn't going to give Botox to Dorathy.

Dorathy's friend Sandra visited with Dorathy often. She would do just about anything to get a laugh out of her or to get her to roll her eyes and shrug her shoulders. These actions from Dorathy made us laugh. It gave us hope that she was constantly making improvements.

Melissa, a minister from Huguenot Road Baptist Church, came in for one of her many visits. As she started to depart after one of her visits, Sandra tried to get Dorathy's hand in the position to wave goodbye to Melissa. Her hand seemed to have a mind of its own, most of the fingers were cupped, and the middle one was protruding. This was definitely not the gesture anyone projected, but it was a comical situation and everyone laughed.

Pull The Plug?

This is a letter I wrote for Dorathy, using Dorathy's words:

UPS Employees

1000 Semmes Ave.

Richmond, VA 23234

May '08

Dear Friends:

Thank you for all the wonderful food you prepared for my family. Thank you for all the flowers, cards, gifts, and most of all I thank you for your prayers and your friendship.

I'll be home soon. I miss you. I am okay.

Love,

Dorathy

Chapter 10

Home

The date, May 21, was a date Dorathy had so looked forward to, and it was finally here. It was a date we had all longed for. All those months in the hospital had not been a picnic for any of us.

Her plight had been very difficult for me; however, I know what I suffered could not have been one-tenth of one percent of what she endured. It broke my heart to see my wonderful daughter struggle and work so hard to do things which had always come so naturally. I wanted so desperately to help her, to make her life a little easier to bear. She still didn't want me to help her do anything, although there were still so many tasks she could not do for herself.

I went to the hospital early in the morning on the day of dismissal to help her dress and get prepared to go home. She was wide awake when I arrived, and was eagerly waiting the return to her home. It had been almost three months since she had left, thinking at that time she would only be away for one night. I was going home with her and planned to stay as long as she would need assistance.

Prior to her dismissal date, she had sent most of her

personal items home; therefore, there wasn't much to pack. I helped her dress and packed the few remaining items that she would be taking home. Dorathy said her goodbyes to the rehabilitation staff, with a mixture of feelings. She had become close to a number of them, and with some she had gotten to be close friends. It was sad to leave, but she was simply elated to be going back to her own home. They were wonderful to her and it was easy to see why they were so great in their chosen profession--they truly cared for their patients.

One of the nurses wheeled Dorathy out of the hospital. When she was outside, a Dunbar armored-van pulled up. Dorathy raised her hand and lifted her thumb as if she was trying to hitch a ride. She really did have a good sense of humor.

As Dorathy departed, everyone expressed delight that she had made so much progress and was now able to go home and continue to recuperate. I think they felt a great sense of pride as Dorathy left, knowing they had done their very best in helping her all they possibly could. She was truly making a world of progress with their help and with the continued help of God.

Of course, it was like Dr. Tate had said during her seminar, "Rehabilitation is like a half-baked cake, and you're only half-way done." There was a lot more work to be accomplished, yet.

Maxine was picked up early from her school that day in order for her to welcome her mom home. Dorathy and Maxine were like two peas in a pod. They were so close, more like close friends rather than mother and daughter. Dorathy was thrilled to be home, and Maxine and I were elated that, finally, she had been released from the hospital to be with us. Again, we thanked God that she had not had to go into a nursing home.

Patrik and Jenn arrived the same day Dorathy was

released from the hospital. I had told them I was going to have a surprise birthday party for Dorathy on May 25th, and they wanted to share her special day with her especially after she had been through so much in the previous three months. Patrik had been extremely dedicated to his sister during her recovery; he visited with her every month.

I had talked with the hospital personnel and had been told that we could use the dining room in the hospital's rehabilitation facility from 1 to 5 p.m. on May 25th, to have a party for Dorathy. When Dorathy convinced the doctors to release her a few days prior to her birthday, we were all happy. Of course, it meant there wouldn't be a birthday party at the hospital, but her friend Larry had planned a party for her and her friends.

The most important point was that Dorathy was again in her own home, and she was constantly making improvements, the smallest of which were always major ones to us. She was, again with her daughter, and I was with my daughter, and granddaughter. We were grateful to God for allowing this to happen.

Dorathy was home, although she needed so much help in every way. Before her release from the hospital, no one knew as to what extent Dorathy's recovery would be. A couple of her closest friends asked me, "What are you going to do with her?"

I replied, "I'm going to take care of her. She's my daughter, and I love her."

They said, "Yes, but this may be forever."

My quick reply was, "Then I will take care of her forever."

Dorathy needed help to feed herself with the feeding tube; her feedings were every four hours. She would take one or one-and-a-half cans of liquid food at each feeding, according to her level of hunger. The cans of liquid feeding were much more convenient than the bag feedings, which some people used. With using the cans, the feedings were much quicker, approximately fifteen minutes, and the patient didn't need to be hooked up to a bag twenty-four hours a day; the patient could more readily move around and work on rehabilitation.

At this time, her inability to climb the stairs made it a necessity for her to stay on the lower level of her home. Her bedroom and bath was upstairs; therefore, the dining room had been converted to her temporary bedroom, complete with the hospital bed. For approximately six weeks, she was limited to sponge bathing. It was fortunate that she had a half-bath downstairs. A lot of help was still needed for her to bath, dress, and undress. Her fingers on the right hand were still not very cooperative, they wouldn't allow her to button or unbutton, zip or unzip her clothing. It took a long time for a sponge bath and for her to dress.

When she was finally attempting to ascend the steps, she had to have assistance to move her right foot up to the next step. Later, she was able to scoot down the stairs step by step while in a sitting position. Getting in and out of bed, covering up, and even turning over was a challenge. She would have to be pulled up and down in the hospital bed. She was later able to use the trapeze bar which had been installed on her hospital bed to pull herself up.

It bothered Dorathy that so many changes had to be made to accommodate her condition. The breakfast room table and chairs were removed from the house and stored; the dining room furniture was moved into the breakfast room to make room for the hospital bed. The door to the half-bath was removed in order for the wheelchair to pass through. Safety bars had to be installed in the shower and other places. A handrail was placed opposite the existing one on the stairway, giving Dorathy a handrail on each side of the stairs.

Home

All area rugs were removed to help prevent her from falling. Ruby, a friend of mine, had a brother, Holt, who had passed away. Dorathy was able to use his wheelchair until her power chair was delivered. Whereas Dorathy was a very petite person, Holt was a big man. The chair was actually too large for her, but it was a life-saver. If she hadn't had it, she would have been in the hospital bed twenty-four/seven.

When the in-home therapy started, the different therapists would come by to visit, and it appeared that they seemed to think it was a social call. Their main objective seemed to be that they just wanted someone to talk to. Dorathy wrote a letter on her new computer to the home healthcare company and to her insurance company. She stated, "In my opinion, the in-home health therapy is for old people who don't plan to go back to work; I am a young person, and I need some additional therapy to help me." She asked me to call the home healthcare company and the insurance company and read to them the letter she had composed. I did so; they both agreed with her.

This is a copy of the letter Dorathy wrote for me to relay to the home healthcare company and her insurance company.

June '08

From my prospective, I think this home healthcare is designed for old people who do not plan to return to a normal life. I have not been overly thrilled with anyone who has been here to date.

It will be two weeks on Wednesday since I was released from the hospital at Johnston Willis. I have only been seen for evaluation and insurance approval. Shouldn't there have been more visits? How soon will out-patient start? Do you know? I want to take advantage of the home therapy, but I am not impressed with it.

I have a list of exercises given to me by JW Hospital.

103

Pull The Plug?

I have not noticed an improvement in my voice. I believe the Vital Stem supplied through Sheltering Arms Physical Rehabilitation Center will be the only thing that will help my voice/throat due to the trauma to my vocal cords from the respirator and trach.

I will be going to outpatient therapy at some point. Who works with the insurance company on a ramp? I would think since the insurance company approved a power chair, they would also approve a ramp. I will have to have a ramp to make full use of the power chair.

How many more sessions are approved for occupational, physical, and speech therapy?

I am asking you to check on this on my behalf. Please keep as close to my thoughts as possible.

The insurance company has approved a power chair for me. It has not been delivered, to date. If one doesn't come soon, a claim will have to be filed for wound care. I have been using a borrowed chair; it is not my size, and it makes my back and bottom hurt due to the fact that it throws me off center.

DSK

During the night, Dorathy would call me using her phone because her voice was still weak. As soon as I would hear the ringing of the phone, I would bound out of bed, in the middle of the night, and dash to her as fast as I could, never knowing if it was an emergency or not. (She had programmed her phone to call me by just pressing one button.)

She received her new power chair on June 4th. Again, this chair was designed especially for her. All the controls were on the left because of the weakness lingering on her right side. Dorathy was delighted to again be able to control her movement from one location to another with just the touch of a button. She no longer had to depend on someone to move her about.

Home

She wanted to take advantage of her new-found freedom by cooking dinner for Maxine the first night. She decided to made spaghetti; I helped her by getting the pans and other utensils out and within her reach. At one point, I stirred the sauce and Dorathy became very upset with me. She yelled at me, "I thought, I was the one making the spaghetti." When this happened, it hurt my feelings, but later I realized this was just one of her attempts to regain her independence.

She also immediately took over the responsibility of paying her bills and managing her finances. Dorathy wanted to get rid of all the clothes and other things she had used in the hospital, as if to wipe away all those memories of her agonizing hospital stay.

Occupational Therapy (OT) had worked with her to retrain her to do her household chores. When I did the laundry, I picked out eight or ten wash cloths and her ankle socks from the dryer. I asked her, "Would you like to fold these?" Dorathy screamed at me as loud as she could saying, "You know I can't do that!" She then started the uncontrollable crying. She was upset that I asked her to do that task. I thought of the request as being part of her continued therapy. OT had her do the same task.

To see her relearning to talk, walk, shower, and dress herself were all major accomplishments. We tend to take all these responsibilities for granted, never thinking about the fact that the brain has to send a signal to a certain muscle to get that task done.

Watching her as she maneuvered her power chair down the ramp that a friend had so kindly built for her was sad. I would watch her and think, this time last year, none of us would have dreamed of Dorathy ever being in a situation such as this.

Gina and Eve came by to visit with Dorathy on June

4th, and Sandra came the following day. Dorathy always had a lot of company, and everyone was so kind to her. That night she called me; I went to her. She wanted to get up from the bed, and I tried to help her. All of a sudden, she started the uncontrollable laughter. When she laughs, she has no control of her muscles. When I tried to hold her up, it was nearly impossible. She and I were approximately the same size. I said, "Dorathy, stop laughing. I can't hold you up to get you in the wheelchair." I didn't realize that at that time she could not control her laughing. She got mad at me and then started the uncontrollable crying. It was a scary situation. If I could not hold her up or manage to get her back into the bed or in the wheelchair, we both might fall to the floor. I was finally, able to get her in the wheelchair, and everything was okay.

Dorathy was still having difficulty with swallowing. Her occupational therapist suggested we string lifesavers on dental floss and make a necklace out of it, thus Dorathy would have it around her neck to keep from swallowing the lifesavers. She could use this to help her learn to swallow again by the sucking and swallowing motion. Dorathy thought this practice really did help her build up the muscles in her throat and mouth; also, she felt it helped the soft palate to begin to do its work. She seemed to enjoy the new exercise, and I do believe it helped her.

A few days later, another therapist arrived to do a physical therapy evaluation. It seemed to be more wasted social time.

Maxine's Godmother and her husband had invited Dorathy and Maxine to their house to spend the weekend. When they arrived to pick them up, they had brought a trailer, in order to transport Dorathy's power chair and the other things that might be needed for their time away from home. Dorathy and Maxine had an enjoyable time, but they were

Home

glad to get back home on Sunday.

Dorathy had agreed to go to Sheltering Arms Physical Rehabilitation Center for evaluation. I was fearful that because I had suggested that she seek help from them, she would not agree to check them out. It was quite a relief when the interview was completed and Dorathy felt so positive about the different ways they had suggested that they could be of help to her. The interview was very helpful, and they were sure their therapy would be beneficial to her. When we returned to her house, she climbed the short flight of six exterior stairs to her porch. As she reached the porch, she started to fall. I immediately put my knee under her, breaking her fall. She fell onto the porch, rather than down the stairs. She and I could not get her to her feet. Dorathy's neighbor is a nurse. She asked me to check with him to see if he could help us. He worked the night shift and didn't answer the door, none of her other neighbors were home. We decided that the only other choice was to call 911. We called them, and they were quickly on the scene. They not only got her to her feet, but they made sure she was comfortable in her house. She only received minor scratches to her right knee; nevertheless, it was a terrifying incident.

A week later on June 13, Dorathy began her day rehabilitation with Sheltering Arms. She was looking forward to getting out of the house and being around other people. She would be working with occupational, physical, and speech therapists. The Van Go Company picked her up and took her to her day's treatment and brought her home each day. Their van had a lift, so Dorathy could go out her back door in her power chair, onto the deck, down the ramp, across the backyard, onto the driveway, and then onto the van's lift and into the van. The driver would then buckle Dorathy's seatbelt and away they would go.

That same day, Dorathy walked up the long flight

of interior stairs to her bedroom with assistance only on a few steps. When she would tire, I would lift her foot a few inches to the next step. She loved the feel of her own bed.

A few days later, Sheltering Arms Physical Rehabilitation suggested that Dorathy needed a special brace on her right foot and leg because her foot kept turning to the side. The new brace enclosed the bottom of her foot and extended up the back of her leg. The brace was ordered, and she was told to wear it every day.

One day in mid June, Dorathy was in her bathroom, and I was in the hall bath. I heard an awful noise; there was no doubt in my mind what the sound was: she had fallen, and I ran to her. There she lay on the bathroom floor, laughing. While seated on the commode, she tried to dress herself, and lost her balance while trying to pull her blouse over her head. It scared both of us. Thank God (again), she wasn't hurt.

The following week Dorathy fell onto the commode. She was a little sore from this fall; however, thankfully, no bones were broken. Her balance was not yet, quite right. She continued to astound her doctors, when she would go in for her check-up, Dr. Wright was amazed that she was doing so well so fast.

Later that day, Dorathy became agitated because I tried to help her fasten her clothes after a visit to the bathroom. It's still so difficult for her to do these small tasks, yet she wants to be completely independent. I do understand that, but when she struggles so hard, it is difficult to just stand aside and not help.

On July 1st, Sheltering Arms Physical Rehabilitation Center worked with me to show me the best way to help Dorathy go up and down a flight of stairs. Afraid she would hurt herself, they didn't like her sliding down the stairs.

Two days later, Dorathy said, "Hey, Mom, watch this." She picked up her tennis shoes, (they were the only type of shoes she could wear to support her right foot); she put the shoe on, and tied it by herself. I had never seen her put her shoe on before, much less tie it. She was always extremely proud of herself when she could show off a new accomplishment, and I was enormously proud to see each one. This was her first week with Sheltering Arms Physical Rehabilitation Center, and she was already making an abundance of progress.

Pull The Plug?

Chapter 11

Goodbye, Mom

On July 4th, we were in her kitchen; I was trying to assist Dorathy with her feeding tube. She was having a difficult time making the liquid food flow through the feeding tube and into her stomach. She was holding the syringe lower than the stomach opening, and this position would not allow the food to go into her stomach.

"Dorathy, why don't you hold the syringe higher to allow the food to drain into your stomach?" I asked.

She became very agitated and yelled at me, "Don't you think I know how to do anything?" She held the syringe higher and the food flowed freely through the tube. It really hurt my feelings for her to yell at me, but I tried to keep in mind the statement that Dr. Tate from Sheltering Arms had made; "A stroke patient's personality can change. They quite often take out their feeling on the person who is closest to them; they want things done for them and they want it done now."

I told her, "Dorathy, I am going to take a nap." I would take a nap when I could. I was so hurt; it was hard to believe she was reacting in that manner. Doing all the different things to help her and being available to do for her around the clock was difficult. Often I would become so exhausted I didn't know if I could continue, getting up early each morning and up at all hours of the night would exhaust anyone. God provided the extra energy.

She told me, "I don't want any more of your friends coming here. They are not coming to see me. They are your friends." My friends had always cared about my family. While Dorathy was in the hospital, she received numerous visits, flowers and cards from my friends. Now, they were forbidden to visit. This new revelation was upsetting. Hardly believing what I was hearing, and informing my friends of the latest predicament was disheartening.

A fellow parish member's brother suffered a stroke. He and Dorathy were in the SICU at the same time. It was ironic to hear the parish member express the daily life of what she and his family were also living through. Their lives and episodes were running parallel to ours. It was hard to believe the two former patients were reacting almost identically.

A person told me about an e-mail Dorathy sent to all her acquaintances thanking them for helping her in so many different ways, but never mentioning all her "mom's" help. It often puzzles me as to why she felt a need to share that bit of info with me. Moms don't need to be thanked during life threatening experiences.

After a nap, I came downstairs, and Dorathy was sitting in her power chair in the kitchen. She said, "Mom, come with me." She led me to her desk and showed me a letter she had written to me. I read the letter. She was mad about the feeding episode. She told me, "Mom, pack your things and leave." This was a real blow; it sucked the life right out of me. I didn't think any mother and daughter could be any closer than my daughter and me. I loved her more than life itself. There wasn't anything I wouldn't do for her. When

Goodbye, Mom

she had her stroke, I quit my job, deserted my church, and left my home and my life in order to be with Dorathy and to care for her twenty-four/seven.

This issue must have had a lot to do with the fact that Dorathy could not always do the things she so desperately wanted to do, so she lashed out at me. I doubt that she really had any intention of hurting me. She was just so driven to recover and didn't want other people doing things for her that she felt she should be accomplishing on her own. All of this affected me a great deal; it was hard to believe my daughter could be so uncaring.

The first month she was in the hospital, I spent hours doing physical therapy, exercising her fingers, hands, arms, toes, feet, legs, and head. This doesn't include all the hours of washing her face, soaking up the ever-flowing saliva, combing her hair, holding her hands, praying, and praying again with and for her. I was devastated by the request for me to leave.

I asked her, "Dorathy, are you sure that is what you want?"

She said, "Yes." I packed my personal items and came home. Needless to say, I felt really hurt, rejected, and depressed. I shared her request with my minister, Fred Spivey, from West End Assembly of God Church. As he had advised me on other matters prior to this, I felt very close to him. He had also visited with Dorathy on many occasions. Fred suggested, "Stay away until she needs something or calls for help." Knowing how badly she needed help, this was difficult for me to do.

While I had stayed with her, she would not allow me in the same room with her when she had visitors. She said, "They didn't come to see you. They came to see me." This seemed to be a strange request coming from my own daughter.

On July 7th, Dorathy had another Barium swallow

113

test and even though she was disappointed, again; she didn't allow the results to get her down.

Dorathy's condition must have been very hard on Maxine. It was hard for an adult to understand, much less a young child of twelve.

I visited with Dorathy for a few minutes. She looked so pretty; more like herself than she had since entering the hospital. She was now walking with a walker most of the time. I had predicted that she would be walking by July, but was told not to tell Maxine because it would just give her false hope; however, my prediction turned out to be very accurate.

———————————

A week later, I picked up Maxine. We enjoyed a movie, while Dorathy went for a check-up with her doctor. The doctor was overwhelmed with the progress Dorathy had made. Toward the end of July, she completed all of her therapy with Sheltering Arms Physical Rehabilitation Center.

When Patrik visited with us at the end of July, they were delighted to see each other. He was totally amazed to see the vast amount of improvements his little sister had made. Patrik's frequent visits were not only helpful to Dorathy, but they were a real gift of peace of mind to me. It gave me a break. It was convenient for Patrik to visit with Dorathy and me since his work as a juror for the Art Institute made it possible for him to travel and work with his laptop computer wherever he was.

The 1st of August, Dorathy asked if I would mind taking Maxine shopping for school clothes, since she was unable to do so. I told her I would love to. We always had fun when we were together, as was the case on that day. She loved picking out her own clothes and was very good at doing so. Going to the mall was relaxing for her. She really needed a break.

———————————

Goodbye, Mom

Dorathy continued to get stronger each day and was still making quite a lot of progress with her exercises. Much tension seemed to be released from her as she went back to work part-time in her home for UPS Freight on August 8th. It had been approximately five and a half months since her stroke. This certainly put a feather in her cap, and she was so happy; another goal reached!

A week later, I tried to work out the difficulties between Dorathy and me. I told her, "If I have offended you by doing or saying something to upset you, I am sorry."

She said, "Just Go-Go-Go!" while pushing me toward her door with the wheelchair. I left. Again, I was very hurt by her uncaring actions and words but she was my daughter, what could I do? If she had been well, it might have been easier to walk away, although in her condition it tore at my heart.

In mid August, I returned to my work as a private duty caregiver/companion. I had been away six months, and I was happy to learn my position with my former client had not been given to someone else. She was a wonderful, lovely, and appreciative lady, she truly felt like family.

The following Sunday, Dorathy ask her friend Larry to drive her and Maxine to Huguenot Baptist Church. The ministers and numerous member of the church had been extremely thoughtful of Dorathy while she was hospitalized. She received stacks of cards from them, laced, with many prayers.

Everyone was happy to see them. Melissa, the assistant minister announced, "The young lady who we have been praying for over the past several months and whose doctors kept saying she'd never make it, is here with us today." It was a very emotional time for Dorathy and for all who had gotten to know her while she was hospitalized. Their visits, prayers, and cards will never be forgotten.

Pull The Plug?

A few days later, I had a freak accident when a wheelbarrow popped up and hit me in the head, as I was unloading bags of dirt from my car. It shocked me, and I immediately drew my hand to my head. When I pulled my hand away it was full of blood. As I washed the area it didn't seem too bad. When Dorathy heard about it, she called to check on me to make sure I was okay. I could tell from the tone of her voice she was worried, and that she really did care about me, even though at times it didn't seem as if she did. I was okay with only a small cut in my hairline and a large goose-egg size bruise.

_____

On August 19th, Dorathy had another Barium swallow test. Finally, she passed it. We thanked God! She could again eat, and we were eternally grateful for this. Her food, however, was limited to applesauce and pudding. She had to eat very slowly. I had thought once she started eating, she could eat anything, but that was not the case. Each week her speech therapist would introduce foods with a little more consistency to them. Still, her liquids had to be thickened. This was a long, long way from what the doctors had all said, "She'll never eat again."

_____

Due to Dorathy's situation, they were unable to take a vacation that year. They had always gone to the beach for a week or two each summer. That year they were only able to take a few day trips. I know they each missed their usual vacation, but they did great dealing with a difficult time.

Chapter 12

Dorathy's Recovery

Because Dorathy was still on a very limited diet, I decided to make her some pizza soup in order for her to have something different to eat. The soup was really different and wonderfully tasty; it had the full taste of a pizza without the crust. It was too thin; though, and Dorathy couldn't consume it. Her soft palate was still not working one-hundred percent. She had to be careful of everything going into her mouth; otherwise, she could choke. That was just too big a risk to take.

Dorathy still could not drive. She called me on the 1st of September saying, "Mom, Maxine is sick. Can you go to the school and pick her up?"

I told her, "Sure, I'd be happy to do so." I picked her up and drove her home. I later took Dorathy to the occupational therapy appointment, and then the three of us had dinner at a nearby restaurant. A few days later, Maxine returned to see the doctor for her checkup; she was fine. I sometimes wonder if the stress from Dorathy's condition contributed to Maxine's health problems. It was a lot for an adult to deal with, much less a young twelve-year old child.

Pull The Plug?

Early in the morning the following day, Dorathy called me. I could tell from the quivering tone in her voice that she was scared and upset; instantly I knew something was definitely wrong. She says, "Mom, can you come over? It's an emergency." This really frightened me. She continued, "My feeding tube is not working. It came out of my stomach."

I quickly replied "I am on my way."

Before I could get out my door, the phone rang again. It was Maxine; she says, "Gran, don't worry about it. I fixed the tube and, it is now working properly. There's no need for you to come over."

What a relief that was; I didn't even know what I would do about fixing the tube once I arrived at their house. I would never have thought that Maxine, at twelve years of age, would even consider repairing the tube. I was proud of her.

In mid September, I took Dorathy some lobster bisque soup. She had enjoyed the soup prior to her hospitalization and I knew she would love to have some. It was so delicious, and she could hardly wait to taste it; however, she was determined to follow her therapist's order of bringing all new foods in to the center in order for her therapist to monitor her eating it, before adding it to her diet. She still had to be extremely careful of all the foods she ate. By doing as her therapist suggested, if she choked, she would have a professional to assist her.

She loved the taste of the soup, but had difficulty eating it and choked. By choking on the soup, it brought out her natural voice, in some way. That night she called me; she was so very excited.

She said, "Mom, Mom, I heard my natural voice today!" I was certain that this was the beginning of the return of her "old" voice; however, that was not yet to be. Knowing her old voice was in her somewhere, I felt sure we would be hearing her speech return to normal just any day. That didn't happen.

_____

A court date had been set for late in September for a six-month hearing on Maxine's temporary custody. Her Godmother had been appointed her guardian. I had kept up with the date and wanted to make sure the custody was kept as temporary. As the court date approached, I called the attorney's office in order to check the court schedule. I wanted to be certain the case was still on the docket. I called Dorathy and told her that the court date for Maxine's temporary guardianship was scheduled for Wednesday.

A few days before the appointed date, I called Dorathy and asked, "Do you want to ride with me to court?

She wasn't nice. She asked, "Why are you going? This isn't any of your business. Why don't you mind your own business?"

I told her, "I didn't mean to get into your business, but I do consider you and Maxine my business. I am only trying to be a supportive and protective Mom and Gran." I had other things I could have taken care of that day, but I felt I needed to make sure Dorathy did not lose custody of Maxine. With Dorathy still unable to do a lot of things, I was fearful the judge might think she was incapable of caring for herself and Maxine; therefore, he might award someone else full custody. That would have been the last straw for Dorathy. I added, "I'll always be here for you, when and if you need me. I love you, Dorth."

My reason for concern of custody was influenced by a court case that took place in Arkansas a few years prior. My niece, Terry, experienced a horrifying situation when she came close to losing her precious daughter, Amy. Terry was terminally ill with chronic obstructive pulmonary disease (COPD), and she had given her best friend temporary custody of her daughter. As Terry became stronger and her health improved, Terry was able to again live at home, and she wanted her daughter with her. However; her (supposed) friend would not allow Amy to return to her home to be with her mother. After a long, drawn out court battle of many, many long enduring months, the judge ordered custody to be returned to my niece. Terry didn't live much longer, but her wonderful little daughter Amy was at her side until Terry took her final breath.

I did not want my daughter and granddaughter to have to endure such a nightmare. Happily, the judge returned full custody of Maxine to Dorathy.

At the end of September, before a planned trip to Branson, Missouri. with my friend Betty, I went to Dorathy's to do some chores for her and some mending for Maxine. We had a nice visit, and later went out for dinner. Some of Dorathy's friends had made plans to assist her while I was out of town. The morning before my departure, Dorathy called me saying, "Mom, I just wanted to call you and tell you to have a safe and happy trip to Branson." It made me feel good that she thought of me. The trip was wonderful.

Dorathy and Maxine were doing great. Dorathy continued to make improvements in her recovery. Every time I saw her, she had relearned another motion. Some doctors have said that there is a real possibility of reconnecting the neurological muscular pathway. It has happened and I thank God for making it possible. I give Him all the praise for each movement and for each breath she breathes.

When Maxine's school choir performed in early October, Dorathy and I took Maxine to her school; it was a beautiful performance. She was just growing up too fast. As I left their home that evening, I told Maxine, "Call me if you want to spend some time with me."

As soon as I walked through my doorway, my phone

was ringing. It was Maxine. She asked, "Is it okay for me to spend the weekend with you?"

I replied, "Sure, would you like to go to the Fall Festival with the ladies from my church and me on Saturday?" She said, "Yes." She went with us, and we all had a great time.

Just prior to us arriving back to Dorathy's house on Sunday, Dorathy fell. I asked her, "Where did you fall?" She says comically, as she points to the spot, "Over there, where you can see my toenails dug up the vinyl floor covering." She again wasn't hurt. Thank God!

Although she has been fortunate each time she has fallen, she continued to fall from time to time. She worked hard to push herself to do all her different exercises to become stronger. Every chance she had, she was on some sort of exercise equipment, working out.

Prior to the 2008 election, I asked her what she thought about the presidential candidates. She said, "To tell you the truth, Mom, I don't like either one of them. Where's Ross Perot when you need him?" It was hilarious coming from her and so unexpectedly. I knew she was not a Ross Perot supporter; but obviously neither was she supporting the other candidates. It tickled me to hear her make that statement, it was so unlike her. Her sense of humor also seemed to be elevated as she recovered from her stroke, (along with her sense of smell, taste, hearing, and sight.) Her doctor said that these senses would return to normal. Dorathy has improved far beyond what the doctors had initially predicted.

The 1st of November, Patrik arrived to check on his "favorite" sister. He, again, was shocked at all the improvements. Changes were still being made every day for the better. Patrik and Dorathy were always delighted to see each other.

Pull The Plug?

Dorathy had an ear, nose, and throat doctor appointment the following day. As we departed her house, the bottom seemed to fall out of all the clouds and the rain poured. Dorathy still had the brace on the right foot and leg. She looked down at her feet and said, "Run, feet, run!" Of course, she could only go so fast. It was so humorous. It reminded me of the Forest Gump movie when Ginny told Forest Gump to "Run, Forest, run," as the mean boys chased him down the long dirt roadway and the braces fell off his legs as he continued to run. Dorathy had retired her arm braces and the left leg brace by this time. Each improvement is a welcomed one. Some days, I would go by Sheltering Arms to watch her work out without her knowing I was watching her. I loved seeing her advance in her skills.

Later in November, she was told she could eat pancakes. She had just recently started eating pizza, and she asked me, "Mom, do you consider pizza as bread?"

"Yes, don't you?" I said.

She replied, "No, I don't because I'm not supposed to eat bread." She continued to enjoy her pizza; she had no problem eating it, and I didn't tell.

My visits with her seemed to improve each time we were together. She now made me feel as if she appreciated all the different things I did or tried to do to make her life a little easier.

In late November, she was told she could eat ice chips. She called me and was extremely thrilled. She said, "Mom, I can eat ice chips!"

I told her, "Dorathy, I'm so happy for you and proud of you."

She said, "Mom, those ice chips were the best things I've ever tasted in my life. They were even better than Starbuck's coffee!" Later she added, "The night after the ice chips were added to my approved foods, I cried and cried. I was so happy to be able to eat ice chips and also happy that my diet was slowly increasing."

Dorathy still had to deal with the feeding tube, but her diet had really expanded. She could now eat a lot, but had to eat slowly. When we would eat breakfast out, her order would consist of two scrambled eggs, grilled catfish, two biscuits with gravy, hash browns, and sliced bananas. She would eat everything on her plate. Her drinks could now be thinner, too. They had been the consistency of honey. Now, they could be thinner as in pectin. If her drinks were too thin, it was more likely they might go down the wrong way and enter her lungs, causing a major problem, such as pneumonia. The latest swallow test was showing continued improvement of the soft palate.

Prior to Thanksgiving, UPS Freight employees notified Dorathy that they would be bringing Thanksgiving dinner for her family, and did they ever deliver! They brought the usual Thanksgiving meal already prepared: turkey and all the trimmings; cases of numerous vegetables, fruits, canned tuna, chicken, cereal, and other items. Dorathy's kitchen counter and the kitchen table were stacked at least three feet high with food of all kinds, and her pantry was overflowing. More food was stored in the bottom of her china cabinet and under her hospital bed. Thanks, again, UPS Freight employees for doing what you do best: delivering.

This Thanksgiving was certainly a day of giving "thanks" to God for the miracle He had performed for us. I was thankful that He allowed my daughter to survive her awful ordeal and that she was continually making more improvements. It was also extremely important that my granddaughter still had her mom and I had my precious daughter. Larry served the wonderful meal for all of us. As we ate, I am sure we were each giving thanks again, thinking about how close we had come to losing a person, who we each loved with all of our hearts.

Along with Dorathy's regular occupational therapy, physical therapy, and speech therapy, acupuncture, and massage treatments were added. During the massage treatment, the masseuse would use their hands as their tools to knead and stroke the muscles and stimulate the blood flow, helping to relax her and reduce the muscle spasms in her right leg.

The chiropractic treatment helped to relax the nerves coming out of her spinal cord. Any slight pressure could compromise an organ or muscle that the nerve feeds. The adjustment allowed the pressure of the nerve to be released and allowed to function to its optimum ability.

Acupuncture is the insertion of needles in key areas to release natural pain killers. This seemed to have sped up her recovery; it relaxed her so much that she would often fall asleep during a session.

When Dorathy completed all her treatments, she would be so relaxed that she would call for an early evening of sleep.

Early in December, Dorathy had an appointment with Dr. Wright for a regular check up. Dorathy asked her, "Would it be okay for me to fly to Arkansas for a wedding?"

Dr. Wright said, "I think it would be okay as long as the plane is pressurized."

Dorathy asked her, "What kind of plane do you think I'm flying on, a crop-duster?" She did fly to Arkansas for the wedding and had a wonderful time.

After that doctor's visit, Dorathy wanted to visit with Dr. Khokhar and his staff. He had helped Dorathy in so many ways. He was instrumental in getting her into the Retreat therapy program. The therapists on his staff were certainly professionals. They knew how to best help, and they wouldn't complain when she would ask for more exercise or therapy as they ended each session.

Dr. Wright suggested that Dorathy should see Dr. Jackson, her neurologist. She wouldn't agree to see him, instead she said, "Why should I see him? He's the one who said I wouldn't live." I think if, it had been me, I would probably have felt the same way, although he did try to help us by making phone calls to the insurance company when we were trying to get her into the Retreat Physical Rehabilitation complex. She continued to exercise in her home, making improvements weekly.

As Christmas approached, Maxine, Dorathy and I decided we wanted to attend the Christmas performance at West End Assembly of God Church, in Richmond, Virginia. It was, as always, a tremendous production. Although, it was tiring for Dorathy to sit for such a long period of time, she enjoyed it too much to complain. We were each in awe.

Finally, on December 8th, after having had the feeding tube for nine months, it was removed. Was she elated! She stated, "It hurt like heck when it was removed, but only for just a second and then it was okay." I had thought after the feeding tube was removed she would automatically go back to her normal eating and drinking routine. That clearly was not the case. She still had to be extremely careful and eat slowly. Her drinks had to be thickened for months after the removal of the tube.

That night, Dorathy and I went to Maxine's school to hear her and her choir sing. She has such a precious little voice; it was an enjoyable evening of music and family.

Dorathy later told me she felt Maxine didn't want her at the school, because she was ashamed of her being on a walker. Trying to assure Dorathy that I didn't think that was the case, seemed to comfort her. I think it helped to be able to discuss this matter.

Pull The Plug?

As part of Dorathy's Christmas, I gave her "a day of beauty." Her hair was cut, styled and colored. Of course a facial is always soothing and relaxing. A manicure and pedicure certainly topped it all. She really enjoyed the pampering she received. She looked great when she emerged from the salon.

The 10th of December was a full day of appointments: acupuncture, chiropractic, speech, occupational therapy, and physical therapy. Afterwards we had dinner at Mulligans and she was delighted to see a number of her old friends there.

A few days later, she called me, asking, "Mom will you come over and pack for Maxine and me to travel to Arkansas?"

I told her, "I have a few errands to run, and then I will be happy to help you." I did some of her household chores, completed the laundry, and then did their packing.

While they were in Arkansas for a wedding, I stayed at their house to care for Lucky, their beautiful Golden Retriever. In order to help out while Dorathy was in the hospital, and after she returned home, Larry kept Lucky at his home. He's a wonderful, well behaved dog, a joy to be with.

Soon after the Arkansas trip, she left her walker outside her bathroom door and entered the bathroom. She called me at my home and asked, "Mom, can you come over? I fell in the bathroom and bumped my head."

I told her, "I'll be right there."

We live approximately twenty minutes away from each other. It scared me to death! With her having had a stroke, I knew her immune system was weak. Things that wouldn't have created a problem before could be major problems now. I was leery of another blood clot. Each time

Dorathy's Recovery

she falls, it frightens me. I am afraid she will break an arm or a leg, either of which would really set her recovery back a long way. Patrik was at my house, and together we rushed to Dorathy's side. When we arrived, she had been helped into bed by a neighbor friend. She had an ice pack on the large, blue goose-egg on her forehead. It looked awful! She was laughing about the situation and seemed to be fine. I was relieved. I joined her in laughing, and we started joking about the goose-egg. Patrik said his final Christmas greetings to us on December 23rd as he departed Virginia, heading for his West Palm Beach home. He spent Christmas with his beautiful Brazilian fiancée in Brazil.

Maxine had not completed all her Christmas shopping, so she wanted to go to the mall. She knew exactly what she wanted to purchase for each recipient and exactly which store would have that particular item. She loved to buy for her mother; however, some of those gifts seemed to have Maxine's name written all over them. We later, enjoyed lunch and a movie.

On Christmas Day, of course, UPS Freight employees would not forget Dorathy and Maxine. Again, a prepared lunch was delivered along with another shipment of every kind of food a person could think of. The UPS elves had really been busy, seeming to have worked all year just preparing gifts for Dorathy and Maxine. Everything you could think of was under their tree. Gifts were piled high and wide, leaving only a narrow path to move through the living room. We had a wonderful, thankful Christmas celebration. Dorathy's friend, Larry, served the dinner. It was delicious; he did a fantastic job preparing the meal.

A few days after Christmas, Dorathy called. "Mom, my ears are bothering me. Will you take me to see my doctor?"

I told her, "Of course, I will." He prescribed some

127

medication and in a few days she was fine.

Her last appointment of the year was with Dr. Martin, her chiropractor. He felt she had made vast improvements. The chiropractic treatment seemed to have aligned the spinal nerves in order to maintain the correct function of the internal organs, lessening her discomfort a great deal.

Chapter 13

Movie

Dorathy and Maxine wanted to see the movie Marlie and Me. I had already seen the movie and it was wonderful. I welcomed the idea of seeing it again. It was about a young couple and their yellow lab, named Marlie.

Near the end of the movie Marlie became ill, and it was evident he would not recover. Dorathy's emotions kicked in. She started crying. As the movie continued, her crying got louder and louder until it was just uncontrollable. She was sobbing so loudly, she could be heard by everyone in the theater. I asked, "Dorathy, do you want to leave?"

She said, "Yes." We left.

When we were outside, she was still crying. She then became upset with me. She said, "I can't believe you 'allowed' me to see a movie like that. You had seen it before, and you knew the dog was going to die." The movie wasn't upsetting to Maxine or me. Dorathy finally settled down.

We drove to their house, and I cooked dinner for the three of us. The evening turned out to be an enjoyable one once Dorathy was okay.

The next day on the radio, the DJ said, "If any of you

are planning to see the movie, Marlie and Me, make sure you take your hankie. My wife and I went to the movie in the Southside Theater last night. A lady was there who became truly upset over Marley's health. She just sobbed and sobbed. You could hear her all over the theater." (The 'lady' was Dorathy.)

A few days later, she called me to come over and do her laundry. Then she got upset because I washed the towels from her bathroom. It was sometimes almost impossible to do things right.

Dorathy decided pool therapy would be good for her, and I agreed. We acquired a membership to the pool at Sheltering Arms Physical Rehabilitation Center. She enjoyed the pool exercises, and it did seem to help her, concentrating on her right leg seemed to be her main objective. The water made it easier for her to move her limbs. She could swim approximately fifteen feet on her back using all her limbs. However, she had to be careful not to get the water in her mouth. Her soft palate had not completely healed, and the water entering the lungs could still cause her problems.

Their pool was beautiful and heated to ninety-one degrees, but it still felt cold in January. Very few people were taking advantage of the pool and I thought that was such a shame.

It was comical; neither of us discussed which swimsuit we would wear to the pool. When we entered the pool, we were dressed alike. We had each worn a black, two piece swimsuit trimmed in white.

That was our first time to swim together since her hospital stay. We had an extremely enjoyable time, playing and working on exercises. As I would lift and bend her right leg, she could slowly swim. Each new accomplishment she made excited me so much, and she was very proud of herself.

Movie

After her chiropractor appointment with Dr. Martin the next day she said, "This treatment really helps me." She appreciated everyone's effort in assisting her.

Dorathy had to continue to be careful of what she ate and drank but it was definitely an improvement over her having to be fed using the feeding tube. I cooked dinner, and we ate together. As I watched her as she ate, tears came to my eyes. I was so happy I still had my daughter and would be able to enjoy many more meals with her.

In mid January, we went swimming again after her speech therapy. We had a lot of fun and were both sore afterwards from the workout. The air was cold when we left the ninety-one degree water. When Dorathy got into the shower, she started calling out for "Mom."I suppose the shock of her going from the really warm water to the cooler air temperature and into the shower must have caused her to hyperventilate. She was gasping for breath. I cupped her mouth and nose with a towel. A bag, which would usually be used in this situation, was not handy. Her breathing slowed to normal. She was okay, although, a little shaken from the scary experience.

The next day, I took her in for her regular doctor's appointment. She continued to improve, and can get in and out of the car completely by herself. Her doctor wrote up orders authorizing Dorathy to increase her work in her home from thirty-three hours to thirty-six hours each week. In February, her hours were increased to a full forty hours, full time.

The doctor also gave her a prescription to take a driver's test (the doctor had to prescribe the test, due to the fact it was administered by the hospital staff) to see if she was capable of driving short distances. She did not take the test right away; she wanted to wait until she felt more capable of driving and making quick decisions. She would quite often become frightened while riding with someone, being afraid when the person in front of her would slow down or stop, thinking the driver was not going to be able to stop in time, or if a car pulled out in front of the one she was riding in, it would scare her. I suppose those senses were also elevated. Maybe that's why she doesn't seem comfortable driving.

In January, I drove Dorathy to speech therapy. I prepared dinner and carried it to her house. She became mad because I delivered the food to them. She said, "You are just trying to run my house by deciding what we will eat. You even turn my silverware upside-down in the dishwasher. You try too hard to help me."

At times it seemed I just couldn't please her, no matter how hard I tried. Times like these were trying to say the least. When I did everything I could to try to make her life a little easier, then she still talked to me as she did. Each time this happens, I hear Dr. Tate's words echoing: "Stroke victims want help and they want it now. They quite often turn against the one person who is closest to them."

Maxine and I thought it was time for us to get out of the house. We went to a movie then returned to take Dorathy to see Dr. Martin for her chiropractor appointment. He was overwhelmed with Dorathy's progress.

The next day, we swam after her speech therapy. She did great exercising. It is easy for her legs to bend in the water. I helped her by bending her right leg in and out, up and down. Dorathy played and exercised at the same time. Her legs seemed almost fully recovered while swimming.

Dorathy continued to work with her speech therapist two or three times a week, her therapist has her repeat different sounds and words to improve her speech. Dorathy followed that up with water exercises and stopped for her chiropractic session on the way to her house.

––––––––––––––

At the end of January, Dorathy asked me to work on her medical and drug bills in order for her to receive reimbursement. I did as she asked. She had all of her medical bills and the forms from her insurance company. I sorted them out, and noted them on the appropriate form.

––––––––––––––

On February 1, we were delighted that Jonathan, her younger brother, returned home safely from a tour of duty in Iraq. He is a career Air Force person and served a number of years with the back-up team for the Thunderbirds. He has also served tours of duty in Afghanistan (three), Iraq (one), and Korea (one). Presently, he is serving a three-year tour in Italy. With Jonathan's military obligations, it was difficult for him to spend as much time with Dorathy as he would have liked; however, they stayed in touch, wherever he might be, and we knew he was with her in thought, prayer and spirit.

Patrik had suggested to Dorathy that acupuncture treatment again might benefit her. She said, "Those treatments really relieve the spasms in my leg and are so relaxing." At that time her spasms were really bad. She was prescribed medication to lessen them.

––––––––––––––

When Maxine and I go out to eat or to a movie, Dorathy cannot always go with us due to her forty hour work week. She is so dedicated to her work schedule. She will comment, "It's time for me to go to the office," as she walks toward her desk or "I can't do that until I get off work." Probably not everyone could work from home, but she is determined to put her time in and to do her work. I'm proud that she is that dedicated. Surely, she missed all her co-workers but she did stay in touch with them.

––––––––––––––

Pull The Plug?

Starting February 9, Dorathy could drink thin liquids with her therapist's supervision. This had been a long time in coming, but she continued to thicken her drinks for months, to avoid the coughing sessions she would sometimes experience, when her drink would go down too fast.

About this time, her leg brace starting bothering her. It rubbed her leg, and it could have caused a blister. She wanted to get it shortened. We went to the doctor's office. He thought she still needed the height of the brace for proper support, and he would not shorten it. However, he did put another strap on it for additional support.

On my birthday, February 20th, Dorathy called me. She sang "Happy Birthday" to me. The song may not have been perfectly sung, but to this mother, it was the most beautiful song I had ever heard. It made me feel great when she would put forth the effort to contact me. She said, "I mailed you a card." I did receive a beautiful card from her and Maxine. Her voice has improved some but she still will not talk with anyone other than me on the phone. She usually corresponds via e-mail.

Three days later, she had a lot of errands to run, in addition to seeing her speech therapist. We had to locate an implement to help her button and unbutton her clothes. The nearby pharmacy had a large selection of medical supplies, and we were able to find the button-hole implement there. She was still having difficulty getting her fingers to do everything she wanted them to do. Her computer, however, was totally a different story; her fingers had mastered that task.

———————

At the end of February, Dorathy's handicapped parking card had expired. She had been given a card for six months. I had to go to her doctor's office to pick up paperwork for a new decal, then by Department of Motor Vehicles (DMV) to pick up the card.

Movie

When Dorathy was first released from the hospital, she would not get a handicapped decal because she said, "I'm not handicapped." Then later she said, "Other people need those handicapped parking spaces more than I do." Finally she decided it could make her life a little less difficult, and she did get the decal.

On February 28th, I found myself looking back. One year prior, Dorathy had surgery and ended up in a coma and quadriplegic. I took her a beautiful bouquet of flowers, some candy, and a card to celebrate the first anniversary. I thanked God for the miracle He gave us in allowing us to be able to continue our lives with her.

She returned to the hospital to visit some of the staff on her anniversary. She also saw one of her doctors. She said, "All the nurses and doctors were shocked to see me walking around when they didn't expect to see me alive."

She told me, "I dreamed a lot while I was in the hospital. I kept having this one dream about you, Mom, over and over again. I would dream I was waking up and there you would be, every time. Then each time when I 'really' woke up, you, again, would always be there."

I told her, "My mom died when I was twenty-one years old. She passed away before I had a chance to fully appreciate her. I hope you know I've always been there when you've needed me, and I always will be."

We took Maxine to the orthodontist for braces. When it was time for her to be fitted, Dorathy stood to go with her and lost her balance, knocking over her walker, and then falling on it. Gosh! Did that scare all of us! Even the doctor came quickly to her rescue. Thankfully she was not hurt at all.

Dorathy was told by her speech therapist to bring

135

some food to eat at her next appointment. We picked up a Caesar Chicken Salad. She was able to eat all of the food without a problem. Her therapist was very pleased with her results. She thought Dorathy was doing great. There had been few foods she tried that she could not eat. When she would eat bread or chesse, it would sometimes stick to the upper part of her mouth. She seemed to have more problems with her drinks than with food.

On the way home, we went by the chiropractor's office. The office was closed, so we treated ourselves to an ice cream treat from the Dairy Queen. She loved the fact that she could now eat ice-cream.

In early March, Dorathy called to say, "Good morning, Mom. I just called to say, Good bye and have a fun and safe trip to Ireland." The tour was a great one. I had looked forward to it for a number of years, and I thanked her for thinking of me. Her short phone calls were so invaluable. Each time the phone rang and I noticed on the Caller ID it was her calling, I thanked God I still had my Dorathia Star. I'm equally thankful she is doing so well in her recovery.

Some days, we did our exercises in her home. She had turned her dining room into a mini gym, with a number of different pieces of exercise equipment and weights. She also added a TV to make the exercise time more enjoyable. The work-outs were great for both of us.

Dorathy asked me, one night, "Mom would you make yagersnitzle for dinner?" That was her favorite German meal, and she hadn't had this meal for over eleven months. I was happy to make it for her. It is made using veal dipped in a mixture of eggs and milk, then breaded and fried. A sauce is made by sautéing onion, bacon, and mushrooms then adding a brown gravy mixture and a small amount of cream. When the sauce is finished, it is poured over the veal cutlets in a serving dish. We usually served it with a salad and French fries.

She loved dinner and certainly ate her share. (I always prepared extra, so she would have some good size portions for later, and she loved that). After dinner, we worked on our exercises, an excellent idea after all that food.

The next day, she decided it was time for a makeover. She asked me to take her to the beauty salon. I was happy to do so. Her hair was cut, styled, and colored. She also had her eyebrows waxed. When they finished, she looked beautiful, like the original Dorathy. The beautification not only helped her outwardly but it also lifted her spirits. I think it was of great importance that she had that time to spend with someone outside of her home. At that time she wasn't getting out of the house much, basically, just for her appointments with her doctors and therapist.

Pull The Plug?

Chapter 14

*The Power to Overcome

At the end of March, Dorathy called and said, "Hey, Mom, I polished my toe nails today and I vacuumed the floor for the first time." She was proud of herself. Each time she accomplishes something for the first time, it simply elates her (and me, too).

With her house newly spiffed up, it was perfect timing when Andy called and wanted to visit with Dorathy. I rode with him. She was really happy to see him and promised, "I will visit your church, H.R.B.C., soon."

———————————

He and I went to The General Nutrition Company (GNC) to pick up a new supply of vitamins and herbs for her. Her doctor had not recommended these, but Patrik was very informed on the subject. Dorathy trusted his recommendations. He had suggested that she add certain herbs and vitamins to the ones she was taking at the time. She thought the homeopathic supplements, used in conjunction with western medicine, had a very positive effect on her healing. The following Sunday, Dorathy asked me, "Would you drive Maxine and me to church?"

Pull The Plug?

I told her, "Yes." I went to her house early on Sunday to assist her in getting dressed. She told me, "I want to go to Andy's church."

I told her, "That's fine. I would take you wherever you want to go." Andy had been ill recently, suffering with a cold and a bad back. I knew he wouldn't be attending church on that Sunday.

So many people from Huguenot Road Baptist Church had visited and prayed for Dorathy while she was hospitalized and after her return home. Dorathy was thrilled to see everyone, and they were delighted to see her. The members of the church all crowded around her as if she was one of their own, hugging her, and telling her how delighted they were that she had recovered so quickly and how pleased she had joined them for church. They, of course, were amazed at her progress. Even though I had told her Andy was ill and wouldn't be at church, she kept looking around saying, "Now, where in the world is Andy?" I think she was just used to him being in his church and she missed him when he wasn't there.

In early April, Dorathy realized she had missed her biannual dental check up, twice. She went in to see our family dentist, Dr. Biggers. He was floored when he saw her, and he couldn't believe she had truly had "The Power to Overcome" the situation she had encountered. He had been shocked when he had first heard of her trauma. He had sent her the most beautiful bouquet of flowers. At times, it didn't seem as though there would be enough hours in our day to do all the different things that had to be done. Rarely did a day pass without an appointment of some sort, and some days there would be four or five. I know it was tiring for her, with the condition she was in. It often got the best of me, but I never let her know. I was just grateful she was still in our lives.

---

*The Power to Overcome

During Maxine's Spring break, Dorathy, Maxine, and some of her friends went to Williamsburg to Busch Gardens. The children loved it and rarely tired, so they were on the go all day, riding all the rides, some of them more than once. I think it did Dorathy and Maxine a world of good to have a day out, although, it did totally wipe her out. She was exhausted when she returned home.

———————

In late April, Dorathy finally took her driving test. She thought she would go in three or four different times, taking part of the test each time before the driving part would be administered.

She did the written part of the test and passed it. After that, she was told to match up the twenty-six letters of the alphabet to the numbers one through twenty-six within a time limit of four minutes. She completed it in one minute and forty seconds. Another test required her to count down from eighty-nine to eighty. They also had her answer a few questions, each of which she answered correctly.

They asked, "What is our current president's name?"; "What is today's date?" and "What time is it?"

She told me, "I cheated on that last question. I looked at my watch."

When those test were successfully completed, Tina, the physical therapist, who administered the test, said, "Okay, let's go."

Dorathy was puzzled and said, "What do you mean?"

Again Tina said, "Let's go."

Dorathy asked, "Do you mean, we're going to drive?"

"No, you are going to drive," Tina answered.

Later in the day, after her friend drove her home, she called me, and I could hear the excitement in her voice. When I answered the phone, she said mischievously, "Mom, this is your daughter, Dorathy. Are you sitting down?"

I sat down. "Okay, Dorth, I am sitting down."

141

Pull The Plug?

She said, so excitedly, "Mom, I drove a car today."

I thought I had misunderstood her. Her voice was not yet back to normal, and sometimes I would not understand what she was saying. She had not been able to drive since the stroke. I didn't know she was going to take her test that day, so I was totally shocked.

Again she said, "Mom, I drove a car today."

I thought maybe it was a simulator from the rehabilitation hospital. I asked, "Was it a simulator?"

She said, "No, Mom. It was a real car with hand controls. It was so great! I drove around in the park, into a neighborhood, and back to the hospital. Initially I was scared to death. Later, I was more relaxed." The UPS Freight employees had hand controls installed on her automobile.

I told her, "Well, that is a giant step for you. I am happy and proud of you!" This news was fantastic. The improvements continued, they had slowed some but as long as she was getting better we were delighted. Needless to say I had to call all of my sisters to share the latest good news with them. They had been my "rock" the past fourteen months.

The following morning early, my phone rang. It was Dorathy, her voice again filled with overflowing enthusiasm. She said, "Mom, I drove a car yesterday!"

I said, "Yes, I know Dorth. You told me yesterday. I'm proud of you and happy for you."

She said, "Yes, I know I told you yesterday, but I'm so excited and happy about it, I just had to tell you again."

Dorothy thought Dr. Martin, her chiropractic doctor, was helping her a great deal with her back and legs. With each treatment, he would massage her back and make adjustments to her spine. He explained to me that each section of the spine controls different parts of the body, and if some part of the spine is not aligned, it can cause pain. Dorothy normally saw him two or three times each week.

*The Power to Overcome

One day as she was completing her session with him, he commented, "I'm proud of your improvements. There has been a big change in you since you first came to see me."

I commented, "Yes. I, too, can see a world of difference in her."

Dorathy added, "Yes, but I still can't play the piano." That comment stunned us. Dr. Martin said, "Oh, I wasn't aware you played the piano. Did you play the piano before the stroke?"

She said with a smile, "No, but I still can't play it."

One of her friends had asked her, "Since you've had your stroke, have you ever had a desire for alcohol?"

Her humorous reply was, "I don't need alcohol because I already walk like a drunk."

Then the friend asked, "Do you ever want a cigarette?"

Dorathy asked, with a playful grin, "Don't you think my voice sounds like the Marlboro woman already, without me smoking a cigarette?"

She had made major improvements in her walking and in her talking. Most complete strangers could now understand her, but she had a long way to go before her walk and her speech would be completely back to normal.

And to think of her neurologist's words a year prior: "She'll never take another step; she'll never utter another word." We are ever so grateful to God, our Father, for each step she takes, for each word she speaks, and for each breath she breathes, even if, at this point she sounds like the Marlboro woman and walks like a drunk.

Another day, she called asking me, "Will you take me to Walgreen's Pharmacy?" I agreed to do so. When we arrived at the store, someone had left their cart outside. The cart was directly in front of my car.

Dorathy took that as an opportunity, "I'm not going to use my walker. I'm going to push that cart."

Pull The Plug?

I sat her walker inside the store's entrance, for her to use when we departed the store.

She pushed the cart up and down every aisle in the store, even if she did not need anything on that aisle. It was almost like Christmas shopping. She had a big smile on her face and acted as if she had finally had her independence completely restored.

At one point, she exclaimed, "This is so much fun!" She handed me her cell phone and asked me to take her picture. She was elated to be so independent.

In early May, Dorathy took a large vitamin. It lodged in her esophagus. It terrified her, but yet she was unable to cough it up or to get it to go down. She was in a lot of pain. Hours passed in this way. Finally, the vitamin dissolved some, and she was able to cough it up. She felt better, but was still concerned that it might cause future problems. She thought she should see a doctor.

Her regular doctor's office was closed; therefore, I drove her to a Patient First clinic, a twenty-four hour medical center. The doctor she saw had never treated her. When he walked into the examination room and saw a young healthy-looking person on a walker he exclaims, "My! And what happened to you?"

She explained, "I had a massive stroke. A blood clot went into my brainstem."

He said, "Oh that could be dangerous."

She asked him, "And how many years in medical school did it take for you to figure that out?"

Everyone laughed. He suggested that she should take some antibiotics for a few days to make sure there were no after effects from the vitamin becoming lodged. She wasn't taking any other medicine at this time, with the exception of the one for the spasms in her right leg.

In June, she wanted to show me, as she lovingly

refers to it, her dog and pony show, her latest accomplishments.

"Look, Mom, I can touch the top of my head with my right hand" as she raises her hand and places it on top of her head. "And look at this Mom… I can walk my hands up the wall." As she would move one hand higher on the wall above the other until she could reach no higher. She would then start over again. I hugged her, and told her, "I love you, and am so very proud of you."

She said, "Mom I didn't do a thing. God did it."

I said, "Yes, I know."

She was so proud of herself and thankful to God, as was I. To people who have never experienced the near death of a child and heard all the doctors repeatedly say, "What you see is all you will get; she'll never get better," these were major accomplishments. Also, these minor tasks probably wouldn't seem of any great importance and wouldn't amount to much. To anyone who is struggling and going through similar situations, I offer you the same advice of the lady in the waiting room and the mystery doctor in the elevator, "Keep your faith most of all, don't give up … death is not the answer; give the person time to heal and then decide what to do. God still heals!" He has The Power to Overcome.

Dorathy, Maxine and I went on our first road trip, since her hospitalization, the end of June. We traveled to Columbia, South Carolina to see Jonathan, my youngest son and Dorothy's brother, and his wife Tracy. He had received orders from the Air Force that he would be transferred to Italy for three years. We wanted to see him before he left the United States.

The trip was enjoyable. It was great to see them. We didn't go out much because the weather was awfully hot. The sun bothered Dorothy's eyes a great deal, they would tear up, and she could hardly see. We were surprised how much hotter the climate was in South Carolina than in Virginia.

It was quiet a relief for Dorathy to get away from home. She loved being with her "little brother" as she affectionately calls him, even though he stands 6'2" and she's approximately 5'2". They've always adored each other. She had not seen him since he had recently returned from a tour of duty in Iraq.

Dorathy hadn't been in a whirlpool since going into the hospital. She decided it was now time to make use of theirs. I ran the water and gathered all her toiletries. I helped her into the tub. She lazily enjoyed the bath, doing some meditating and relaxing for approximately forty-five minutes. But when it was time to exit the tub, she was unable to do so. We had a lot of trouble getting her out. Finally, I put some towels on the floor; she bent over the edge of the tub. I picked up her feet and legs and lifted them over and out of the tub.

She said, "I won't do that again," as she laughed. She was then able to dress and do her hair.

I was so thankful to God for allowing Dorathy to still be with us and to accompany us on this trip.

She had made the statement, "I feel I'm in jail. I live at home. I work at home. I rarely get to go out." I think the trip helped her; although the trip there and back was extremely tiring for each of us.

When we returned home, she said, "I'm so glad to be back in my own bed. While at Jonathan's, I kept thinking I was rolling out of bed."

———————

After seventeen months, Dorathy still fell from time to time. She fell onto the treadmill once but said she didn't need to see the doctor; her neck was just a little sore.

As I watched her do all her exercises, it made me

sad. It is still quite a struggle for her to move from one piece of exercise equipment to another. It is a major job for her. Other people, who have not been through a similar situation, might think if she can walk with only a walker or quad cane, she should be able to do any exercise; however, after all this time and all the improvements she has made, she still has to put a lot of effort into every goal. Her latest fall left her in the floor of her walk-in-closet. She again said, "I wasn't injured to the point of needing a doctor." She didn't seem to want to see a doctor unless it was a real necessity. I suppose she felt she had had her share, after seeing so many of them.

Dorathy went for another drive at the end of July. She said, "It felt better this time. I did much better. With the right hand getting stronger, I am able to change gears more easily and right turns feel better."

Dorathy also enjoyed her ride at the grocery store in their power shopping carts. I think it makes her feel more independent to be able to shop for her own groceries. Later we stopped at GNC to restock her vitamins and herbs. We exercised when we returned to her house.

It is wonderful that she was still making improvements. Some doctors had said while Dorathy was still in the hospital that all her improvements would come in the first six months. She was exceeding that. Other people would tell me their relatives were making progress in their 11th year.

At one time she was having a lot of difficulty moving the right leg. It didn't want to bend, and sometimes it was still stubborn; however, there had been improvement by this time. Her leg spasms seemed to be less frequent and her right arm was stronger.

At the end of July, she said, "I'm going to check on getting back into rehabilitation." Thinking that was a wonderful idea, I encouraged her to do so. Sometimes, her exercises left me feeling depressed. She pushed herself so hard.

Pull The Plug?

To watch her crawl from one piece of equipment to another was sad. Still feeling down when I stopped to fill my car with gas at the local 7-11 store, I noticed a van pull in and park in front of the store. For some reason my attention was drawn to it and I continued to watch. Slowly the back passenger side door opened, a ramp came down and out rolled a power chair with a man in it. He had no arms and he had no legs. The chair evidently was controlled by voice.

This really touched me. I thought of the old cliché about the man who complained about not having shoes until he met the man who had no feet. I was delighted to still have my daughter.

Later in the week, I picked up some three pound weights for Dorathy to use with her home exercise program as she had asked of me. She walked around the kitchen without her walker in August. Her leg was much improved. It not only bends at the knee, but also up and down at the ankle. In mid August, Dorathy told me, "I'm so excited about my leg bending. I'm going to take a picture of it and send it to everyone."

At the end of August, Dorathy fell onto her walker as she was getting out of bed. Her mouth was cut and swollen. It appeared that she bit the inside of her mouth along the cheek line between the two rows of teeth. When I was questioning her about her fall, she said, "Well, I'll tell you, if you are not planning to write a book about it." We both laughed.

In September, Dorathy and I joined the Sheltering Arms Physical Rehabilitation Fitness Program. Maxine was too young to use their equipment. We had hoped she, too, could benefit from the workouts.

Later that week, Dorathy drove roughly ten miles. She drove to Maxine's school, around the school, and back home. The drive totally exhausted her. She said, "I felt like I had driven four or five hours." When she returned home,

*The Power to Overcome

she had to have a nap. She was totally wiped out. Since then I don't believe she has had a desire to drive at all.

Pull The Plug?

Chapter 15

Today

Today … 26 months after her surgery, God is still watching over Dorathy as she continues to improve.

She has started her speech therapy, again. Denise, her new speech therapist, who is with Sheltering Arms Physical Rehabilitation Center is so dedicated to teaching and helping Dorathy to speak more clearly. With only three weeks of the new therapy, her improvement is absolutely remarkable. Her voice is much louder and clearer.

The spasms in her right leg are not as severe as they were. She does take medication to relieve the spasms. That is the only medication she takes, other than the vitamin supplements.

She can bend her right leg enough to ride an exercise bike and to walk some. The majority of time, she leaves her walker behind and relies on the quad cane to assist her. Some of the times, she leaves them both sitting and continues on her way, unassisted. At times, Maxine now hides her mother's walker and cane, to encourage her to walk on her own.

Dorathy can drive but does very little of it. She

doesn't yet feel confident enough to drive a lot. At this time, she has to have a licensed person riding with her. I believe Dorathy is afraid she might not be able to react fast enough in a case where time might be of the essence to avoid an accident.

Her employer, co-workers, and friends continue to be so supportive. Her job of forty hours a week is still accomplished in her home.

Her daughter, Maxine, is almost fourteen years old. She has grown into a beautiful, independent young lady, who has certainly been tested these last couple of years. Maxine now does a lot of the cooking, laundry, and other household chores. She assists her mom in many ways while still being a teenager.

I continue to help Dorathy and Maxine. We go to the gym three nights a week. The exercises have benefited all three of us. She is still simply elated when she is able to perform a movement or exercise that she wasn't able to succeed at before.

I drive Dorathy to her speech therapy appointment twice a week and to other appointments and to run her weekly errands. She is now able to get in and out of an automobile completely unassisted, including retrieving the seat belt and fastening it, and opening and closing the car door.

Chapter 16

Special Thanks

Dorathy's friend, Jacqie, was certainly a dedicated and devoted friend to her. She and her family were by Dorathy's side as soon as they heard of the predicament she had encountered. They were constantly at the hospital to support Dorathy.

Jacqie's husband, Andrew, even snuck into the Surgical ICU while Dorathy was still in a coma. She recalls exactly what he told her, "At this point, God is your only hope, and you, also, need to be praying along with us."

After the hospital's chaplain delivered the mind boggling news to Maxine about her Mom's true condition, Carson, Jacqie's and Andrew's daughter, kept Maxine company. Carson and Maxine were the same age and had shared some classes. They were dear friends; Carson acted like a young adult trying to console and comfort her best friend.

For months, Jacqie prepared and delivered food to Maxine. Dorathy wasn't able to eat since she still had her feeding tube. While Dorathy was in the hospital, Maxine spent most of her time with Jacqie and her family in order for Maxine to stay in her own school.

Pull The Plug?

    Furthermore, when Dorathy returned home from the hospital, Jacqie and Andrew were constantly "on call," any time, day or night. Dorathy could and would call them for help with numerous tasks. Never did they say, "Sorry or it's too late or it's bad timing." They were always willing to help in any way they could. Words cannot convey how wonderful these precious people were. May God richly bless them.

    Teresa and Tim, dear friends of Dorathy's and Maxine's, also helped out beyond the call of friendship. In the three months Dorathy was in the hospital and after she returned home, they became like family. Their numerous visits were very important.

    Prior to Dorathy's return home, Teresa went to Dorathy's house and gave it a thorough cleaning. She had her mom, Sarah, come by and shampoo all the carpet.

    When Dorathy returned home, Teresa and Tim would come to visit. She would spend hour after hour helping Dorathy with her exercises, bending and raising her arms and legs. In the meantime, Tim would make any repairs needed, take care of odd jobs, or would mow the yard. Teresa also helped with Maxine's care, while Dorathy was still in the hospital. Some of the time she would spend the night with her in order for Maxine to be more comfortable in her own home. She taught Maxine to sort and launder her clothes. Tim and Teresa also ran lots of errands for Dorathy. Better friends could not be found. They were so loving and dedicated; there must be extra stars in the halos waiting for them.

    The UPS Freight employees could not have been more understanding, caring, or helpful at any point. They were always there. They were with us from the day of Dorathy's surgery, when she went into the coma, and even now. All the visits, flowers, cards, gifts, and most of all-the prayers, were very much appreciated.

    The fact that a schedule was made for those who

Special Thanks

wanted to prepare and deliver all the delicious food to our family was certainly beyond the call of friendship, but, it was gratefully appreciated. All the supervisors and employees who took their time to help transport Dorathy to hundreds of therapy sessions, doctor's appointments, chiropractic sessions, massage treatments, or just simply came by for a visit or said a prayer... you helped make life for her easier to bear at a really rough time in her life.

The delivery of the laptop to the hospital and setting it up for her, when she could hardly move her hands was another Godsend. It gave her hope and incentive for the future. The words, "Thank you" would never be enough to express my feelings and appreciation to each of you.

A special thanks to John for all the phone calls he made to keep Dorathy out of the nursing home. I know there were ways, too numerous to mention, he helped, that I know nothing of. That is when we see someone's true self; when they're doing what's right, not when they're doing something for someone to see it being done. I shall always be grateful to you as I know Dorathy is.

There were so very many other people who were extremely kind, dedicating their precious time, their work, and so much more to help Dorathy. Each gesture, each thought, and each prayer was exceedingly appreciated. Thank you, thank you, and thank you!

Pull The Plug?

Chapter 17

Ministers/Churches

I am very grateful, and want to thank each person who prayed a prayer for Dorathy; God surely heard those prayers, and He answered them by allowing Dorathy to stay with us and for her to be a testimonial for Him.

Dorathy always had an abundance of cards, flowers, gifts and visitors coming into the hospital. In order to make room for future deliveries, she sent flowers home weekly. She cherished each expression of concern. To this day, she keeps every card in a special basket near her desk and her mail still includes cards each week.

The church of my sisters, Loretta and Linda, the Gardner First Baptist Church in Gardner, Kansas, sent cards and prayed for Dorathy weekly. They were super supportive during her long stay in the hospital and after her return home. I visited their church in October and met some of the members who had been praying for Dorathy. Reverend Ken Porter announced to the congregation, "The mother of the young lady, Dorathy, who had the massive stroke and who we've been praying for all year, is with us today along with all of Dorathy's aunts. He continued, "Pat has reported to me that Dorathy is doing great. Improvements are remarkable; she is now talking some and is walking with the assistance of a walker. She still has her feeding (Peg) tube and the leg brace, but she's looking forward to the day she can give those up. Dorathy is getting stronger each day."

The members of Huguenot Road Baptist Church were also extremely caring and loving. Some members, who themselves had difficulty walking those long hospital corridors, never let that get in the way of visiting and praying for Dorathy three or four times each week. Prayers and cards from Huguenot Road Baptist Church were received constantly. Reverend Melissa, Reverend Bert, and numerous other members of the church became like family during the long enduring months of Dorathy's hospitalization. Each time she would see them approaching, a big smile would appear on her face; she always enjoyed their visits immensely.

My church, West End Assembly of God, was also with us from the start. Reverend Bill Martin was with us for prayer prior to the surgery. Members of the church had prayed with me on Sunday before the surgery. Carol, an acquaintance and fellow parishioner, tried to assure me many times by saying, "Everything is going to be just fine." Reverend Fred Spivey and Reverend Bill Martin visited with Dorathy on many occasions; they also anointed her with oil. (The anointing of oil is to help the person being anointed to heal). Our Sunday school class prayed for Dorathy so often and so sincerely, I sometimes felt guilty asking for prayer for her again each week after giving a praise report.

Ministries/Churches

Churches Praying for Dorathy

Gardner First Baptist Church
Gardner, Kansas
Reverend Ken Porter
(Sisters Linda's and Loretta's Church)

_____

West End Assembly of God
Richmond, Va.
Reverend Bill Martin, Reverend Fred Spivey
and Reverend John Hershman, Senior Minister
(My church)

_____

Huguenot Road Baptist Church
Richmond, Va.
Reverend Bert Browning and
Reverend Melissa Fallen
(Andy's church)

_____

Set Free Church
Warm Springs, Va.
Reverend Mike Puffenberger
(Leeoma's sister's church)

_____

Cornerstone United Methodist Church
Jonesboro, Arkansas
Reverend Tommy Toombs
(My sister, Retha's church)

_____

Pull The Plug?

The Community Church Assembly of God
Rock Creek, Ohio
Reverend Bryan Wright
(My Sister, Vernice's, Church)

The 700 Club, Christian Broadcasting
Virginia Beach, Va.
Reverend Pat Robertson

Asbury Memorial United Methodist Church
Chesterfield, Va.
Reverend Derrick Parson
(Neighbor Phyllis's church)

Janke Road Baptist Church
Richmond, Va.
Reverend Lance Yost
(Marilyn's church)

Oak Grove Baptist Church
Richmond, Va.
Reverend Bernard Whitlow
(Dorathy's friend's church)

Buford Road Baptist Church
Richmond, Va.
Reverend Tony Kahout

Ministries/Churches

In Dorathy's words
A Letter to Gardner First Baptist Church
(My Sister's Church)

1/8/2009

Hi Folks,

I wanted to update you on my progress as so many of you continue to make my day. Almost a year ago something happened to me that changed my life, and the lives of others were changed forever. Not a week goes by that I don't receive cards. They help; as the prayers did and still do! Almost a year ago I went into the hospital to have a "simple procedure" to fix a heart Arrhythmia (WPW). I'm not sure at what point my Aunt Loretta and/or Linda asked you for your prayers. I suffered a massive stroke at the brainstem. According to the Doctors who looked at the MRI, I wouldn't be "checking out" as intended. In fact, I wouldn't be anything more than remain in a vegetative state for the rest of my life. I remember looking around wondering why everyone was making such a big deal of things. When I heard them say "We are afraid of her brain swelling," I got scared. I prayed and prayed. I've never been very religious. I have always believed in Jesus Christ; was baptized as a child; knew the Bible (Bible drill) from church camp functions. I don't remember if it happened before the coma or after, a family friend snuck into my room (I was in ICU--no visitors). He told me that the only thing that could help me at that point was God. I prayed and prayed again. The next thing I realized, my brothers were there, too! Mom... I told her it would be a "simple procedure" out of the hospital the next day. This looked like it would take longer. My "li'l" brother (that stands 6'2"), was crying. He started asking me questions, but the Doctors had already told us that I was

Pull The Plug?

"Locked-In" (only able to blink my eyes) and one eye was doing its own thing anyway. He asked me yes/no questions. Then he knew he was onto something when he would get a decent response. "Is your hair red?" No response. "Is your hair brown?" BLINK. We played this game for a while, and then he wanted to show the Doctors, as they were having discussions about me being an organ donor and that I had a "Living Will." My family told the Doctors that at some point I had moved my leg. His response was, "Just a reflex; what you see is all you'll get." Jonathan asked me if I was hungry. BLINK ,BLINK, BLINK. He ordered them to give me a feeding tube. Mom had been "exercising" me even although she got NOTHING back. Due to the trauma from the tubes down my throat and the overall stroke, I've been unable to speak; but I've come so far! I used to use a cardboard "communication" board that people would have to point to the letters and wait for my "BLINK." I can speak now and be understood by most. Still don't "do phones." My left side returned 100% in May; still working on some things on my right. I walk with a walker still. Though have done the four prong cane, my ankle, knee and hip need to come round more. My right hand is good; in fact I'm again using it to type. There are some limits; but gains have been made! I am a skeptic by nature. But as I said, I've always believed. The gospel has always been my favorite. If I didn't believe before…modern-day miracle, no doubt! I just hope I'm forgiven when I walk back in the hospital and punch the Doctor. I plan to tell the judge it was just a "reflex." I returned home with my daughter in May and Mom brings over your cards from her house. Don't stop the prayers please, THEY WORKED. They got the "Right Doctor" in charge to take over. Don't EVER doubt who is really in charge! Thank everyone, please, for the cards! I've kept every one of them. DSK

This experience has changed our lives and the lives of others, forever. It has drawn our family closer and also closer to God. Of course, I do not know what God has in store for Dorathy. I only know he has given us a miracle, for which I shall always be grateful. Throughout this entire ordeal, Dorathy has been the strongest and most courageous person I've ever known. Enduring all the trials and trepidations could not have been an easy task. She was wired for courage.

I believe He placed Dorathy on this earth to show people that miracles still exist in our modern day world and created her to work for Him, to be a testimonial for Him.

For anyone who might find themselves in a dilemma such as we experienced, I strongly suggest you take the advice of the mystery lady (in the SICU waiting room) and the doctor (in the elevator).

"Give her time, see how she does and then decide. There's no hurry."

If a person has a family member who is ill and suffering, don't take death as an answer. Don't give up. Only God knows how many days or years a person has left.

If only one person, who reads our story, decides to give their loved one more time and that person lives, I feel it will have served as the purpose for sharing our situation. I am thankful I listened to those two wise people. Had I not, I would have wondered for the rest of my life if things could have been different and if I made the right decision. I am delighted I can look at my daughter from across the room or across the table and smile at her as she returns the smile … not realizing my smile is because I'm immensely grateful she's still in our lives to exchange those smiles of much gratitude.

I could not save Dorathy's life by all the things I did or tried to do for her. I did put everything I had to give into helping her all I could, as any mother would do. God is the one and only one who brought her back. I give him all the praise, while still praying and thanking Him each day. I often think of her in a coma; how many times daily I would stroke her hair, wash her face, and say her name over and over again, unwilling to give her up. All those trials were worth it and then some.

This isn't all He wrote. This is not the end of our story. It is the beginning of a closer walk with our God. I believe He has already written that Dorathy will fully recover. We just must wait and again give Him time to do "His thing" in His own way. "Thank you, Lord for not taking my precious daughter.

To Remember Me

The day will come when my body will lie upon
a white sheet neatly tucked
under four corners of a mattress located in a hospital;
busily occupied with the living and the dying.
At certain moments a doctor will determine that my brain
has ceased to function and that,
for all intents and purposes, my life has stopped.
When that happens, do not attempt to instill
artificial life into my body by
the use of a machine. Don't call this my deathbed.
Let it be called the bed of life and let
my body be taken from it to help
others lead fuller lives.
Give my sight to the man who has never seen a sunrise,
a baby's face or love in the eyes of a woman.
Give my heart to a person whose own heart has caused
nothing but endless days of pain.
Give my blood to the teenager who was pulled
from the wreckage of his car,
so that he might live to see his grandchildren play.
Give my kidneys to the one who depends
on a machine to exist from week to week.
Take my bones, every muscle, every fiber and nerve in my
body and find a way to make a crippled child walk.
Explore every corner of my brain.
Take my cells, if necessary, and let
them grow so that, someday a
speechless boy will shout at the crack
of a bat and a deaf girl will hear
the sound of rain against her window.
Burn what is left of me and scatter the ashes
to the winds to help the flowers grow.
If you must bury something, let it be

Pull The Plug?

my faults, my weaknesses and
all prejudices against my fellow man.
Give my sins to the devil
Give my soul to God.
If, by chance, you wish to remember me,
do it with a kind deed or
word to someone who needs you.
If you do all I have asked, I will live forever.

Robert N. Test, Author
Printed with permission

Pull the Plug?

By Patricia A. Smith

Pull The Plug?

Wolff-Parkinson-White Syndrome

What is the heart's normal condition?
In a normal heart, electrical signals use only one path when they move through the heart. This is the atria-ventricular or A-Vnode. As the electrical signal moves from the heart's upper chambers, the atria, to the lower chambers, the ventricles, it causes the heart to beat. For the heart to beat properly, the timing of the electrical signal is important.

What is the Wolff-Parkinson-White Syndrome?
If there's an extra conduction pathway, the electrical signal may arrive at the ventricles too soon. This condition is called Wolff-Parkinson-White syndrome (WPW). It's in a category of electrical abnormalities called "preexcitation syndromes," and is recognized by certain changes on the electrocardiogram, which is a graphical record of the heart's electrical activity. The ECG will show that an extra pathway or shortcut exists from the atria to the ventricles.

Many people with this syndrome who have symptoms or episodes of tachycardia, rapid heart rhythm, may have dizziness, chest palpitations, fainting or, rarely, cardiac arrest. Other people with WPW never have tachycardia or other symptoms. About eighty percent of people with symptoms first have them between the ages of eleven and fifty.
How is this syndrome treated?
People without symptoms usually don't need treatment. People with episodes of tachycardia can often be treated with medication, but sometimes such treatment doesn't work. Then they'll need to have more tests of their heart's electrical system.

The most common procedure used to interrupt the abnormal pathway is radiofrequency or catheter ablation. In this, a flexible tube called a catheter is guided to the place where the problem exists. Then that tissue is destroyed with

Pull The Plug?

radiofrequency energy, stopping the electrical pathway. Successful ablation ends the need for medication. Whether a person will be treated with medication or with an ablation procedure depends on several factors. These include the severity and frequency of symptoms, risk for future arrhythmias, and patient preference.

American Heart and Stroke Association

Printed by permission

NINDS Locked-in Syndrome Information Page

What is Locked-in Syndrome?
Locked-in Syndrome is a rare neurological disorder characterized by complete paralysis of voluntary muscles in all parts of the body except for those that control eye movement. It may result from traumatic brain injury, diseases of the circulatory system, diseases that destroy the myelin sheath surrounding nerve cells, or medication overdose. Individuals with Locked-in Syndrome are conscious and can think and reason, but are unable to speak or move. The disorder leaves individuals completely mute and paralyzed. Communication may be possible with blinking eye movements.

Is there any treatment?
There is no cure for Locked-in Syndrome, nor is there a standard course of treatment. A therapy called functional neuromuscular stimulation, which uses electrodes to stimulate muscle reflexes, may help activate some paralyzed muscles. Several devices to help communication are available. Other treatment is symptomatic and supportive.

What is the prognosis?
While in rare cases some patients may regain certain functions, the chances for motor recovery are very limited.

What research is being done?
The NINDS supports research on neurological disorders that can cause Locked-in Syndrome. The goals of this research are to find ways to prevent, treat, and cure these disorders.

National Institute of Neurological Disorders and Strokes

Printed by permission

Pull The Plug?

Life Net Health Media Relations Contact: Doug Wilson
Transplant and Donation Statistics: 757.609.4468

Donation and transplantation save lives. There is a critical shortage of organs in Virginia and nationwide. Three Virginians die each week waiting for a life-saving organ transplant that doesn't come in time.

One donor can save nine lives through organ donation (heart, liver, pancreas, 2 kidneys, 2 lungs, and small intestine), enhance more than fifty lives and restore sight to two people through eye and tissue donation.

To be an organ, eye, and tissue donor, the most important thing you can do in Virginia is document your wish at DonateLifeVirginia.org or at a DMV office.

DonateLifeVirginia.org is the new website in Virginia where you can sign up online to be an organ and tissue donor. The process is free, simple, and secure. It only takes a few minutes to sign up online.

DonateLifeVirginia.org works in partnership with the DMV's organ donor program. If you sign up to be an organ, eye, and tissue donor at the DMV then your information will be transferred to DonateLifeVirginia.org. (Everyone who signed up as a donor at the DMV in the past is already in the DonateLifeVirginia.org database.)

Your designation at DonateLifeVirginia.org or your driver's license or a donor card is a legal document and your wish will be honored. Family permission is no longer required in Virginia, except in the case of a minor.

More than 110,000 people are currently awaiting an organ transplant in the U.S.; more than 2,900 of those are in Virginia.

On average, eighteen men, women, and children die each day waiting for a lifesaving organ transplant in the U.S.

About 28,000 organ transplants take place in the U.S. each year and on the average 700 of those are in Virginia.

Life Net Health is the non-profit agency that handles organ and tissue donation in Virginia. Life Net Health coordinates the recovery and placement of organs, teaches the public about donation, and handles a bereavement program for donor families.

Life Net Health coordinates the recovery and placement of organs in Virginia, teaches the public about donation, and handles a bereavement program for donor families.

Life net Health has a volunteer team of more than 300 people in Virginia that help educate the public about donations. Donor families and transplant recipients participate in speaking engagements, health fairs, and events.

To learn more about organ and tissue donation or to volunteer, call Life Net Health at 1-866-728-3738 and visit LifeNetHealthOPO.org.

Life Net Health helps to save lives and restore health for thousands of patients each year. We are the world's most trusted provider of transplant solutions, from organ procurement to new innovations in bio-implant technologies and cellular therapies—a leader in the field of regenerative medicine, while always honoring the donors and healthcare professionals who allow the healing process.

Life Net Health

Printed by permission

Pull The Plug?

Order Form

Use this convenient order form to order additional copies.

Pull The Plug?

Please Print:

Name: _____

Address: _____

City:_____ State:_____

Zip: _____

Phone:(_____)_____

_____ Copies of book @ $15.95 each $_____

Postage and handling @ $4.00 per book $_____

VA residents add 5% tax $_____

Total amount enclosed $_____

Make checks and money orders payable to
Patricia A. Smith and mail to:

Patricia A. Smith
8048 Buford Commons
Richmond, VA 23235

pattya46@verizon.net

Pull The Plug?

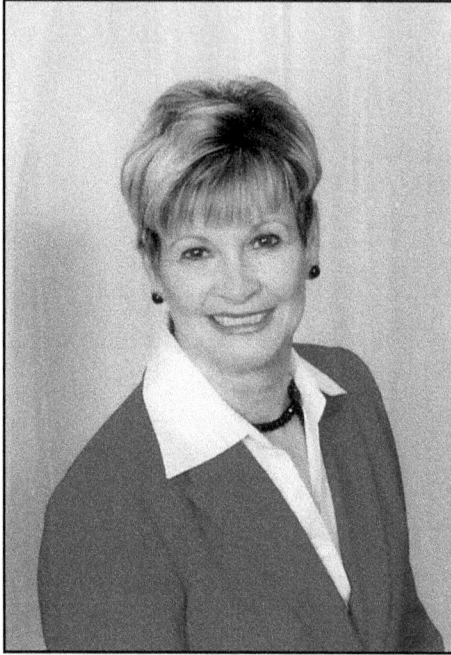

Photo courtesy of SEARS

Patricia Smith resides in Richmond, Virginia. She is originally from Arkansas and attended Austin Peay State University, where she majored in Business Administration. After marrying a career military man, she and her family spent many years living in Europe, where the children were educated. Patricia worked for the European Division of Max Factor in Belgium, Germany, and Holland. She is the mother of Dorathy, Patrik, and Jonathan and the proud Gran to her only grandchild, Maxine. Along with writing, Patricia enjoys photography, oil painting, reading, dancing, boating, traveling, her family, her friends, and her church.

www.ingramcontent.com/pod-product-compliance
Lightning Source LLC
Chambersburg PA
CBHW052004090426
42741CB00008B/1543